MODERN
URINE
CHEMISTRY

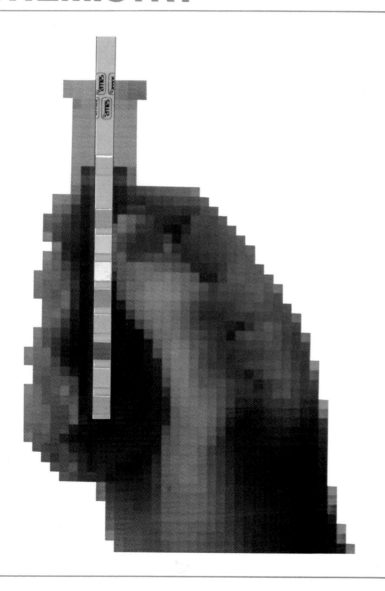

TABLE
OF CONTENTS

PREFACE

This book is designed to provide the reader with a review of basic laboratory procedures useful in routine urinalysis. The methodology and purpose of selected basic tests are presented; reference values are given and the clinical significance of abnormal results discussed.

In addition, some procedures not commonly included in routine urinalysis are described, together with new convenient methods for bacteriuria detection and specific gravity determinations. The intent is not only to provide condensed technical information on urinalysis procedures, but also to give the reader a comprehensive view of the extent to which the routine urinalysis and supplemental procedures can supply clinically valuable information about the health status of the patient.

This revised edition incorporates and updates information pertaining to routine urinalysis since this original book was published.

Recent advances in technology has resulted in the improvement of existing urine testing products; the introduction of new tests; and the introduction of automated and semi-automated instrumentation to the field of urinalysis testing.

Photomicrograph credits to: Rachel Lehman, BS, MT (ASCP) and Wake Forest College, Bowman Gray School of Medicine, 1982.

"Modern Urine Chemistry" is provided as a service to the medical community by AMES, Division of Miles Laboratories, Inc., Elkhart, Indiana 46515, U.S.A.

August 1976, AMES COMPANY

Fourth Printing

Revised 1982

RENAL STRUCTURE AND FORMATION OF URINE

1.

A basic background about kidney structure and urine formation is an aid to understanding urinalysis and test interpretation.

Analysis of urine is used for two purposes. One is to ascertain the existence of body disturbances, such as endocrine or metabolic abnormalities in which the kidneys function normally and, therefore, excrete abnormal amounts of metabolic end products specific for a particular disease. The second purpose is to detect intrinsic conditions that may adversely affect the kidneys or urinary tract. Diseased kidneys cannot function normally in regulating the volume and composition of body fluids and in maintaining homeostasis. Consequently, substances normally retained by the kidney or excreted in small amounts may appear in the urine in large quantities and substances normally excreted may be retained. Structural elements, such as red blood cells, leucocytes, cells from the urinary tract, and casts from the diseased kidneys may appear in the urine.

Components of the genitourinary tract are shown in Figure 1. Normally there are two kidneys, two ureters, one bladder and one urethra.

NORMAL GENITOURINARY SYSTEM

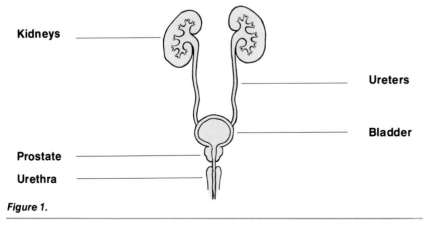

Kidneys

Ureters

Bladder

Prostate

Urethra

Figure 1.

ANATOMY OF THE KIDNEY

The gross anatomy of the kidney is shown in Figure 2.

The functional unit of the kidney is the *nephron.* There are approximately one million nephrons in each kidney. (Figure 3).

Each nephron consists of a *glomerulus,* which is essentially a filtering system, and a *tubule,* through which the filtered liquid passes. As liquid moves through the tubule, various changes occur: certain constituents are reabsorbed by the cells lining the tubule, and other substances are secreted into the lumen for eventual excretion. On the average, nearly all of the water that passes through the glomerulus, with the exception of a liter or so, is reabsorbed by the tubule.

Each glomerulus consists of a network of capillaries surrounded by a membrane *(Bowman's capsule)* which continues on to form Bowman's space and the beginning of the renal tubule. The *afferent arteriole* carries blood from the renal artery into the glomerulus where it divides to form a capillary network. These capillaries reunite to form the *efferent arteriole,* through which blood leaves the glomerulus. The blood vessels then follow the course of the tubule, forming a surrounding capillary network.

The tubular portion of each nephron has several distinct structural and functional segments. The uppermost portion, continuous with the glomerulus, is the *proximal convoluted tubule,* followed by the *thin-walled segment* and the *distal convoluted tubule* respectively. The decending limb of the proximal tubule, the thin-walled segment, and the distal tubule form a loop known as the *loop of Henle.*

KIDNEY

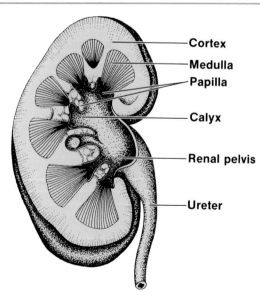

Cortex
Medulla
Papilla
Calyx
Renal pelvis
Ureter

Figure 2.

NEPHRON

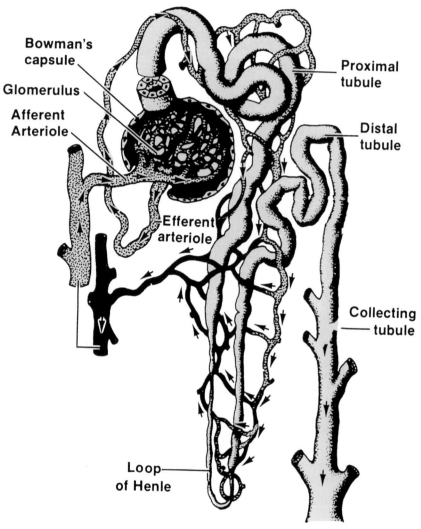

Figure 3.

The *distal convoluted tubules* from several nephrons drain into a *collecting tubule*. A number of these coalesce to form the *collecting duct*. The collecting ducts then join together to form the *papillary ducts*. The latter empty at the tips of the papillae into the calyces which in turn drain into the renal pelvis. Urine passes from the pelvis of the kidney down the ureter and into the bladder, where it remains until voided.

FORMATION OF URINE

The kidney should be thought of as a highly discriminating organ which maintains the internal environment by selectively excreting or retaining various substances according to specific body needs. Approximately 1200 ml of blood flow through the kidneys each minute. This represents about one-fourth of the total blood volume. The blood enters the glomerulus of each nephron by passing through the afferent arteriole into the glomerular capillaries.

The capillary walls in the glomerulus are highly permeable to water and the low molecular weight components of the plasma. They filter through the capillary walls and the closely adhering membrane of Bowman's capsule into Bowman's space. From here the plasma ultrafiltrate passes into the tubule where reabsorption of some substances, secretion of others, and the concentration of urine occurs.

Many components of the plasma filtrate, such as glucose, water, and amino acids, are partially or completely reabsorbed in the proximal tubules, while in the distal tubules more water is absorbed and potassium and hydrogen ions are secreted. The loop of Henle and the system of collecting tubules are the principal sites where the urine is concentrated as a mechanism for conserving body water. (Figure 4).

FORMATION OF URINE

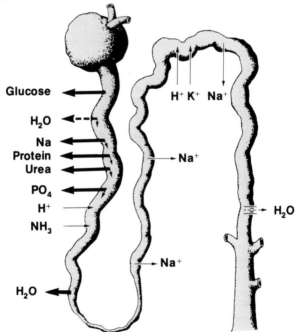

Figure 4.

12

THE BASIC URINALYSIS

2.

Urinalysis is routine for many patients seen in the physician's office or medical clinic and for every physical examination. The testing is usually repeated annually or as frequently as the physician deems necessary. It is one of the most useful procedures available to the physician as an indicator of health or disease, especially in the areas of metabolic and renal disorders.

Urinalysis is frequently run on the patient's urine at the time of hospital admission and is often repeated to evaluate health status while the patient is hospitalized. The steps involved in routine urinalysis can be divided into three basic categories. A fourth procedure—detection and semiquantitation of bacteriuria—can now also be done easily in the urinalysis laboratory. The major observations and determinations appropriate to each category are listed in the following outline.

PHYSIOCHEMICAL CHARACTERISTICS
- Color
- Volume
- Appearance
- Specific Gravity

CHEMICAL EXAMINATION
- pH
- Protein
- Glucose
- Ketone
- Bilirubin
- Occult Blood
- Nitrite
- Urobilinogen
- Ascorbic Acid

MICROSCOPIC EXAMINATION
- Epithelial Cells
- Casts
- Crystals
- WBC's
- Bacteria
- Yeast
- RBC's
- Non-Bacterial Organisms

BACTERIAL SCREEN
- Gram Stain
- Colony Count

A recent innovation, N-MULTISTIX-SG,® allows the specific gravity of a urine to be measured chemically on a strip rather than by the conventional methods.

STANDARD PROCEDURE

Most testing is done on a random specimen of urine, freshly voided by the patient. The specimen is collected in a clean, dry container and examined within one hour to avoid changes or deterioration in the urine. If the specimen is to be kept more than one hour before the analysis, it should be refrigerated at 5° C.

In the laboratory, the first procedure is to note the physical characteristics of the urine; the second is to measure the specific gravity; and the third is to run a series of chemical tests. A 10—15 ml aliquot of the thoroughly mixed urine specimen is centrifuged and the residual sediment resuspended in ¼—1 ml of urine for microscopic examination.

The remainder of the urine specimen should be saved until all procedures are completed so that any of the tests may be repeated, if necessary, or other special tests can be performed, if so indicated.

CHEMICAL TESTS

Chemically-impregnated reagent strips are available for rapid determinations of urine specific gravity pH, protein, glucose, ketones, bilirubin, hemoglobin, nitrite, urobilinogen, and ascorbic acid. These strips are used in basic urinalysis and have virtually replaced older, more cumbersome methods. In addition, other reagent strips, chemical tablets, selectively-treated slides, and simplified culture tests are available for special determinations. Instrumentation, such as the CLINI-TEK® can process reacted reagent strips to allow standardization of the results.

Detailed descriptions of all of the procedures outlined in the routine urinalysis described above are presented in the following chapters.

COLLECTION OF URINE

3.

In order for urinalysis to be meaningful, the urine must be properly collected. Improper collection may invalidate the results of the laboratory procedures no matter how carefully and skillfully the tests are performed.

CONTAINERS

Containers used for collecting urine are quite variable in type, but regardless of type, they must be capable of being *cleaned and thoroughly dried* before specimens are collected. Without these initial safeguards, test results will be less meaningful, if not meaningless.

Because the requirement for scrupulous cleanliness of urine containers involves considerable expense in hospitals where hundreds of specimens are collected daily, disposable specimen containers are gradually replacing traditional glass bottles. Disposable containers of plastic or coated paper are available in many sizes and are provided with lids for covering the specimen to reduce bacterial and other types of contamination. Special pliable polyethylene bags are available for collection of urine from infants and children not toilet-trained.

URIN-TEK® disposable collection system (Fig. 5) is available for use in collecting, storing, transporting, and testing specimens of urine. The system consists of a flat-bottom paper collection cup, a plastic 15 ml tube with a plastic snap-cap and self-adhesive identification label. Disposable tube holders are available for handling ten tubes at a time. Wire carrying racks for transporting 20 tubes are also available. The patient voids directly into the paper cup, the specimen is transferred to the URIN-TEK tube, and the plastic cap is applied to prevent contamination or spillage of the specimen. After the label is filled out and attached, the specimen is ready to be transported and analyzed. Specific gravity can be run directly in the URIN-TEK tube if a urinometer is used. By using the convenient reagent strip, many of the chemical tests can also be performed directly in the URIN-TEK tube thus obviating the need of additional laboratory glassware. It also eliminates transferring and relabeling of the specimens with the concomitant increased risk of errors in identification.

Large, wide-mouthed plastic or glass containers with screw-cap tops are used for cumulative collection of urine over a long period of time.

These bottles should be kept refrigerated or should contain an appropriate chemical preservative.

When urine is to be examined and cultured for bacterial content, the specimen must be obtained under aseptic conditions (as discussed later in this chapter) and collected in a sterile container. The collection receptacle may be either a sterilized glass container or a sterile plastic disposable container. In either case, the receptacle should be equipped with a tightly fitting, sterile cap which is left in position until the actual time of urine collection and replaced immediately afterward.

URIN-TEK® SYSTEM

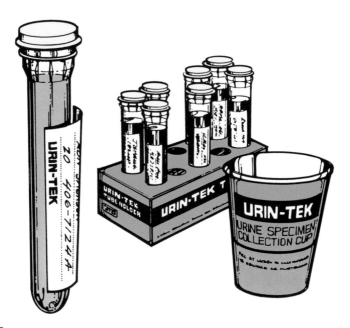

Figure 5.

METHODS OF OBTAINING SAMPLES

A freshly voided urine specimen is adequate for most urinalysis except the bacteriologic examination. The patient should be instructed to void directly into a clean, dry container or into a clean, dry bedpan and then transfer the specimen directly into an appropriate container. Specimens from infants and young children can be collected in a disposable collection apparatus, consisting of a plastic bag with an adhesive backing around the opening to fasten it to the child so that he voids directly into the bag. All specimens should be covered immediately and brought, without delay, to a storage place or laboratory. If a urine specimen is likely to be contaminated with vaginal discharge or menstrual blood, then a clean-voided specimen must be obtained using the same procedures described below for collecting specimens for bacteriologic examination.

METHOD OF OBTAINING A CLEAN-VOIDED SAMPLE

The procedure most commonly used for obtaining urine suitable for bacteriologic examination is the collecting of a clean-voided midstream specimen. Bladder catherterization and percutaneous suprapubic aspiration of the bladder may be used, but only in very rare and unusual circumstances. Collection of a clean-voided specimen is the method of choice unless specific contraindications exist. To avoid contamination of the voided specimen by organisms in areas adjacent to the urethral meatus, this area must be cleansed thoroughly before the patient voids. To avoid contamination of the specimen with organisms often harbored normally in the distal urethra, the initial stream of voided urine which clears these organisms from the urethra is discarded and the subsequent midstream urine is collected.

A satisfactory technique for the female consists of spreading the labia and cleansing the area with three gauze sponges moistened with green soap solution. The washing is accomplished by making a single *front-to-back motion* with each of the sponges in sequence. One is used to cleanse the area on one side of the meatus, the next used for the other side, and the third directly across the meatus. One dry sponge is then used with a single front-to-back motion to remove the soap and dry the area. While the labia are still held apart, a small amount of urine is passed into the toilet or bedpan to be discarded; then a midstream specimen is collected in the sterilized container which is immediately closed with its sterilized cover.

A comparable technique is used for males by retracting the foreskin of the penis, cleansing the glans and particularly the area surrounding the meatus, with three sponges moistened with green soap solution, and wiping off with a dry sponge. With the foreskin still retracted, a small amount of urine is passed into the toilet or bedpan to be discarded. From the subsequent midstream urine a specimen is collected in the sterilized container.

For infants and children who have not been toilet-trained, a sterilized disposable collection apparatus can be used to obtain specimens after the perineal region has been suitably cleansed.

TYPE OF SAMPLE

The concentration of urine varies throughout a 24-hour period depending partly on the patient's water intake and partly on his activities (Table 1). Various solutes may appear in greater or lesser amounts at various times of the day—glucosuria appears more often after meals, proteinuria may occur following activity or assumption of the orthostatic (upright) position, and hemoglobinuria may follow severe exertion. The number of bacteria in the urine of a patient with a urinary tract infection varies greatly throughout the day. In general, a more concentrated urine is preferred for testing rather than a dilute specimen. Therefore, the first-voided morning urine, which is the most concentrated, is the best one for routine anaylsis. Often it is not practical to obtain the first morning specimen, and in such cases a randomly voided specimen of lesser concentration is usually obtained. Therefore, the effect of the concentration of a sample, as measured by the specific gravity, should be considered in the interpretation of the results.

Routine tests and any other tests performed on a random sample of urine are qualitative in nature. At best, only the concentration of a substance in the specimen tested can be measured but never the total amount being excreted unless the urine is collected over a precisely measured period of time. For example, two random specimens are tested for proteinuria. One may show a heavy concentration of protein and the other only a slight amount. If the first specimen is a very concentrated sample and the second a very dilute sample, the actual total amount of protein may be greater in the second. A 24-hour specimen may provide a more representative sample in these cases.

Table. 1.
COLLECTION OF URINE

FIRST MORNING SPECIMEN
- Most concentrated
- Bladder incubated

Best for:
- Nitrite
- Protein
- Sediment overview

Note: Formed elements may lyse or disintegrate if urea splitting bacteria are present.

RANDOM SPECIMEN
- Most convenient
- Most common

Good for:
- Chemical screen
- Microscopic examination

SECOND-VOIDED SPECIMEN
The first morning specimen is discarded. The second specimen is collected and tested.
- Reflection of blood glucose
- Formed elements intact

POSTPRANDIAL
- Good for glucose
- Collected after a meal

2-Hour volume
- Good for urobilinogen and glucose

24-Hour volume
- Necessary for true quantitative results

PRECAUTIONS IF URINE IS NOT EXAMINED WITHIN ONE HOUR

When urine is delayed for periods longer than one hour before analysis, special precautions must be taken both to avoid deterioration of chemical and cellular elements and to prevent multiplication of bacteria that may be present in the collected urine, with resultant alteration in urinary constituents. Bacterial multiplication regularly occurs in urine specimens that remain at room temperature for several hours. Bacteria may utilize any glucose in the urine, and the urea-splitting organisms convert urea to ammonia, producing an alkaline urine. In addition, casts decompose in an alkaline and/or hypotonic urine, after several hours, and red blood cells may be lysed. Marked changes in pH may also affect other cellular components.

Refrigeration at 5° C is often the only precaution needed to preserve the urine for routine analysis. However, chemical preservatives may be necessary when specimens cannot be refrigerated, as when a patient transports a specimen from home to office or laboratory, or when the specimen is sent in by mail, or when a specimen is routed about a hospital or large laboratory. Preservatives should always be used cautiously, however, since a preservative suitable for some test procedures may interfere with others.

The selection of a specific preservative must be determined by the procedures to be performed. Preservative tablets that produce formaldehyde, such as Urokeep®, Cargille Urinary Preservative Tablets, and

19

Kingsbury-Clark Urine Preservative Tablets, are available and are much more convenient to use than liquid formaldehyde. These tablets do not interfere with the usual chemical and microscopic examination. Formaldehyde retards the deterioration of casts and cellular elements. Toluene is one of the best and most frequently used preservatives. Thymol, as crystals or in solution, and boric acid, 0.8% solution are also useful preservatives.

Too much preservative may interfere with the urinalysis. Thymol in amounts of 0.1 gm/dl may give false positive reactions for albumin in some test procedures. Formalin may give a false positive reaction for glucose with certain test procedures. Urine to be analyzed specifically for glucose is best preserved with benzoic acid. For determination of urine pH and titratable acidity, any preservative that will affect pH or acidity must be avoided.

Obviously no chemical preservative should be added to urine specimen that will be used for bacteriological examination since the preservative will destroy the viability of most of the bacteria that may be present. It is preferable to make such culture tests immediately. Otherwise the specimen should be refrigerated at 5° C, and culture tests done within eight hours.

APPEARANCE OF URINE

4.

The first observation usually made on a urine specimen is its appearance. Initially, this is done unconsciously and unthinkingly by virtue of just handling the specimen. However, careful attention to details and correlation with past experiences can provide useful clues to the presence of many substances in the urine specimen. For example, a dark color may indicate a concentrated urine; a pale color, dilute urine; a reddish-brown color, blood. A turbid specimen may suggest an alkaline urine. A trained observer is able to gain important clues about the urine simply by its appearance.

COLOR

The color of the urine is affected by many components, e.g., concentration, food pigments, dyes, blood, etc. The intensity of the color of normal urine is dependent on the concentration of the urine. The yellow or amber color of a normal urine is due to the presence of a yellow pigment, urochrome.

The color of urine changes in many disease states because of the presence of pigments that do not normally appear. Bile pigments may produce a yellow to yellow-brown or greenish color; the porphyrins produce a dark brown-red color upon standing; hemoglobin gives a reddish-brown color. Melanins cause urine to turn a brown-black color upon standing. Alkaptonuria is identified by urine that turns dark brown or black upon standing. The urine may assume many different colors following the ingestion of various dyes, foods, and drugs.

ODOR

Normal, freshly voided urine has a characteristic aromatic odor which is believed to be due to the presence of volatile acids. Urine that has been standing for any length of time develops an ammoniacal odor which is due to the decomposition of urea in the specimen.

The urine of patients with diabetes mellitus may have a fruity odor due to the presence of acetone. The urine of patients with urinary tract infections may be foul-smelling, especially when the infecting organism is a coliform bacillus. Certain foods such as asparagus may impart a characteristic odor. Although the urine may have many characteristic odors, as a rule, the odor of the urine is not considered to be of special diagnostic significance. Perhaps the classical exception would be the mother who was instrumental in identification of phenylketonuria by noticing a peculiar odor to her child's diaper.

TURBIDITY

Normal, freshly voided urine is usually clear or transparent, but also may have a cloudy or turbid appearance due to the presence of phosphates and carbonates if the specimen is alkaline. This cloudiness will disappear when the urine is acidified. A pinkish turbidity frequently indicates the presence of urates. Abnormal turbidity of urine may occur with urinary tract infections, but this is usually due to the alkalinity rather than to the actual number of bacteria or leukocytes present.

SPECIFIC GRAVITY

5.

The specific gravity of urine indicates the relative proportions of dissolved solid components to the total volume of the specimen. It reflects the relative degree of concentration or dilution of the specimen. Knowledge of the specific gravity is needed in interpreting the results of most tests performed in routine urinalysis. Under appropriate and standardized conditions of fluid restriction or increased intake, specific gravity measures the concentrating and diluting abilities of the kidney.

EXPECTED VALUES

Specific gravity of urine may range from 1.003 to 1.030, but usually remains between 1.010 and 1.025. Specific gravity is highest in the first morning specimen and is generally greater than 1.020. A specific gravity of 1.025 or above in a random normal urine specimen indicates normal concentrating ability. The kidney's ability to concentrate can be measured by the so-called concentration test. This test is run by withholding all fluids after the evening meal, as ordered by the physician. Urine passed during the night is discarded, and the first morning specimen is tested. A specific gravity of 1.026 or higher is considered normal.

Dilution tests are less useful than the concentration tests since they provide less information about renal function. They are also potentially hazardous to the patient. In conditions such as Addison's disease they are usually inadvisable. The procedure requires the patient to take a suitable water load, usually one liter during a 30-minute period; following this, normal patients will excrete at least one urine specimen with a specific gravity less than 1.003 in the next hour or so.

CLINICAL SIGNIFICANCE

LOW SPECIFIC GRAVITY

Diabetes insipidus, a disease caused by the absence of, or impairment to, the normal functioning of the antidiuretic hormone (ADH), is the most outstanding and severe example of loss of effective concentrating ability. This disease is characterized by large urine volumes of low specific gravity. Specific gravity in such cases usually ranges between 1.001 and 1.003.

Low specific gravity may also occur in patients with glomerulonephritis, pyelonephritis, and various renal anomalies. In these cases, the kidney has lost its ability to concentrate the urine because of tubular damage.

HIGH SPECIFIC GRAVITY

Specific gravity is high in patients with diabetes mellitus, adrenal insufficiency, hepatic disease, and congestive cardiac failure. It is elevated whenever there has been excessive loss of water, as with sweating, fever, vomiting, and diarrhea.

Abnormally high amounts of some of the urinary constituents, in particular glucose and protein, increase the specific gravity producing measurements of up to 1.050 or more in the urine of some patients with diabetes mellitus or nephrosis. The specific gravity increases 0.004 for every 1% glucose in urine and 0.003 for every 1% protein in solution.

FIXED SPECIFIC GRAVITY

Urine with a fixed low specific gravity (approximately 1.010) which varies little from specimen to specimen is known as isothenuric. This condition is indicative of severe renal damage with disturbance of both the concentrating and diluting abilities of the kidney.

DETERMINATIONS

Specific gravity is a measurement that indicates the density of the urine. It is a number derived from the ratio of the weight of a given volume of urine to the weight of the same volume of water, under standardized conditions.

$$\text{Sp. Gr.} = \frac{\text{weight of urine}}{\text{weight of water}}$$

Water has a specific gravity of 1.000. Since urine is a solution of minerals, salts, and organic compounds in water, the specific gravity is greater than 1.000. The relative difference reflects the degree of concentration of the urine specimen.

DIRECT METHOD—URINOMETER (FIGURE 6)

The specific gravity of urine can be determined with a urinometer. This is a weighted, bulb-shaped instrument that has a cylindrical stem which contains a scale calibrated in specific gravity readings. This instrument is floated in a cylinder containing urine. The depth to which it sinks in the urine indicates the specific gravity of the urine, which is read on the urinometer scale at the junction of the urine with the air.

The urinometer is calibrated to read 1.000 in distilled water at a specific temperature, indicated on each instrument. There is a change in the specific gravity of 0.001 for each 3°C above and below this temperature. For precise work, temperature corrections must be made on the readings. For example, correction for error is required if the urinometer reads 1.004 in distilled water; .004 must be subtracted from each reading. Correction for temperature is accomplished by adding (or subtracting) .001 for each 3°C above (or below) the calibration temperature. Corrections are also recommended when glucose or protein are present. It is recommended that .003 be subtracted from urinometer readings for each 1000 mg/dL of glucose or protein. The urinometer requires large urine volume and is cumbersome to perform.

URINOMETER

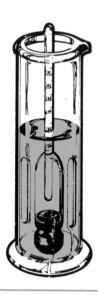

Figure 6

DIRECT METHOD-FALLING DROP (FIGURE 7)

Like the urinometer (hydrometer), the falling drop method is a direct measurement of specific gravity. With this method, a drop of urine is dropped into a series of columns, each filled with solvent mixtures of increasing steps of known specific gravity. If the drop of urine comes to rest after its initial momentum is dissipated and then neither rises nor falls, the specific gravity of the urine is the same as the solvent mixture of the particular column. This procedure for determining specific gravity is not "new." Graded series of mixtures of xylene and bromobenzene, chloroform and benzene, and bromobenzene and kerosene have been employed. Prior to development of the Refractometer, a distinct advantage of such techniques was that only a few drops of sample were required for the determination. These techniques, however, have never achieved popularity for use in routine urinalysis—probably because of the obvious time requirements in setting up such a system.

The procedure utilized for specific gravity determinations with the Ames CLINILAB® instrument is the "falling drop method." As indicated, this is a direct measurement method of specific gravity and the procedure is specific and thus more accurate than refractometry; it is also more precise than hydrometers. Unlike the graded series of mixtures described above, the CLINILAB® uses a silicone base oil with a controlled value of specific gravity and viscosity in a specially designed column. This column was developed to measure the time required for a precisely measured specimen drop to fall a distance defined by two optical gates (lamp-phototransistor pairs) mounted one above the other in a temperature-controlled column, filled with the water-immiscible fluid of a slightly lower density. The light beams from these lamps travel through the column oil and strike phototransistors located on the opposite wall of the column. The specific gravity column is equipped with an overflow system that permits sample fluid (urine) to drain continuously into a liquid waste container without losing any of the column fluid.

A drop of urine dispensed into the column oil by the CLINILAB® pipette will break the beams of light as it falls through the oil. Breaking the upper beam starts an electronic timer; breaking the lower beam stops the timer. The falling time is measured electronically and computed into specific gravity units.

FALLING DROP METHOD

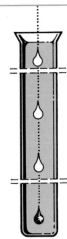

Figure 7

INDIRECT METHOD—REFRACTIVE INDEX (TS METER)

An indirect method of measuring specific gravity is refractometry, i.e., American Optical® Total Solids Meter. (Figure 8) The TS Meter measures the refractive index of the solution. The refractive index is the ratio of the velocity of light in air to the velocity of light in solution. The refractive index varies with, but is not identical to, the specific gravity of urine.

Although the AO® TS Meter measures refractive index of a solution, scale readings have calibrated in terms of specific gravity, refractive index and total solids.

The AO® TS Meter requires calibration daily. The TS Meter is temperature compensated between 60°F-100°F. The scale reads in increments of 001 from 1.000-1.035. Urines of specific gravity less than 1.017 are read more accurately using a refractometer than are urines of specific gravity readings above that level.[4]

TS METER

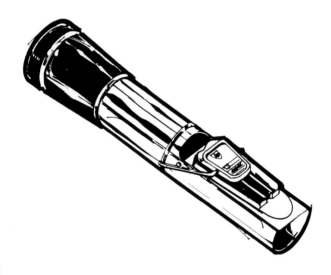

Figure 8

INDIRECT METHOD—REFRACTIVE INDEX (DIGITAL URINOMETER, BIOVATION, INC.)

Another instrument that indirectly measures specific gravity by refractometric methodology is Biovation's Digital Urinometer®, (Figure 9). Approximately 4 mL of urine is required for operation. The principle of operation is the same as the TS Meter. The Digital Urinometer reads specific gravity from 1.000 to 1.040 in increments of .001. The velocity of the light passing through the cuvette of the instrument is compared to the velocity of light passing through a known standard solution.

Carry over of specimens is not usually a problem but occurs more where there is a substantial difference (>.020) between specimens. It is recommended that these specimens should be retested for greatest accuracy.

Two calibration solutions are required, Hi-Cal and Lo-Cal. As with all instruments, routine maintenance and calibration checks are required. Controls and standards are recommended.

MODEL 300
DIGITAL URINOMETER

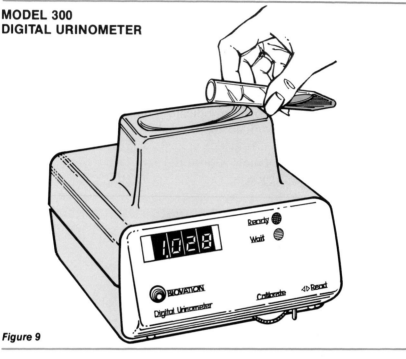

Figure 9

INDIRECT METHOD—IONIZATION OF POLYELECTROLYTE

The newest indirect method of estimating specific gravity is the Ames Specific Gravity Reagent Strip method. The N-MULTISTIX® SG is not the first indirect method for measuring specific gravity. It is, however, the first method in the disposable, convenient reagent strip format and the first to be directly combined with the existing reagent strips used in the clinical laboratory.

The specific gravity reagent area has three primary ingredients impregnated into the reagent paper:

- a polyelectrolyte-polymethylvinyl ether/maleic acid, partially neutralized
- an indicator, bromthymol blue
- buffers

The principle of the specific gravity reagent area is based on a pKa change of certain pretreated polyelectrolytes in a relation to the ionic concentration.

The reagent area has been impregnated with a polyelectrolyte (long chain molecule). This particular polyelectrolyte (polymethylvinyl ether/

28

maleic acid) is different because it contains acid groups (carboxylic acid) that dissociate releasing charged ions as shown below. Ions are charged particles. The charge could be positive or negative.

RCOO–H = Carboxylic Acid

$RCOO–H = RCOO^- + H^+$

Summarizing the principle, in the specific gravity reagent area of the multiple strips the polyelectrolyte, polymethylvinyl ether/maleic acid, is sensitive to the number of ions in the urine specimen. When the concentration of electrolytes increases (high specific gravity) in the urine, the pKa of the polyelectrolyte in the reagent strip is decreased; thus, the pH decreases. The bromthymol blue indicator changes colors from blue-green to green to yellow-green indicating the pH change caused by increasing ionic strength (increasing specific gravity) and is empirically related to specific gravity values (Figure 10).

Color block quantitation is:

1.000
1.005
1.010
1.015
1.020
1.025
1.030

PRINCIPLE OF N-MULTISTIX® SG

SPECIFIC GRAVITY: pka CHANGE/IONIC CONCENTRATION

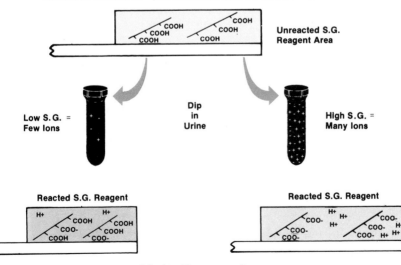

A Surface Phenomenon On
Cellulose Fibers

Figure 10

OSMOLALITY

6.

Osmolality of the urine is a more exact measurement of urine density than specific gravity. Osmolality depends on the number of particles or solute in a unit of a solution, whereas specific gravity depends on both the quantity and the precise nature of the particles in solution. Large dense particles such as protein, sugar, and intravenous dyes increase urine specific gravity disproportionally more than the osmolality. Because the determination of specific gravity is so simple and easy to perform, this measurement is generally performed in the routine laboratory analysis and serves quite adequately for the majority of specimens. Whenever a more precise measurement is indicated, osmolality of the urine can be determined.

Measurement of osmolality of a solution is a measure of the number of osmols in one kilogram of solution. Thus, it is a measure of the number of particles in a given weight. This is often confused with osmolar solutions; osmolarity is a measure of the number of particles in a given volume of solution, osmols per liter of solution. Results are expressed as milliosmols (1 osmol = 1000 milliosmols). The osmolality and osmolarity of relatively dilute solutions, such as urine, are practically identical and the differences are generally neglected in routine laboratory examinations.

REFERENCE VALUES

Normal kidneys are capable of diluting and concentrating urine from a minimal range of 40 to 80 mOsm/kg water during a water diuresis to a concentration of from 800 to a maximum of 1400 mOsm/kg water with fluid deprivation. The normal range of urine concentration for a patient on a normal fluid and food intake is from 500 to 850 mOsm/kg water.

PLASMA URINE OSMOLALITY RATIO, OSMOLAL CLEARANCE, AND FREE WATER CLEARANCE

Evaluation of the concentrating and diluting ability of the kidney can progress beyond routine clinical measurements to determinations of the ratio of plasma to urine osmolality, the osmolal clearance, and the free water. The ratio of plasma/urine osmolality measures the concentrating ability of the kidney and normally ranges from 3.0 to 4.7. The osmolal clearance reflects the ability of the kidney to conserve or excrete water. It equals the ratio of the urine osmolality to the product of the plasma osmolality multiplied by the rate of urine flow in ml/min. The free water clearance is a better expression of this kidney function. Free water clearance equals the urine flow, in ml/min, minus the osmolal clearance.

$$\text{Free water clearance} = \text{urine flow} - \frac{\text{urine osmolality}}{\text{plasma osmolality}} \times \text{urine flow}$$

When "free" water is excreted, urine osmolality is less than plasma osmolality; when water is being retained, urine osmolality is greater than plasma osmolality. Free water clearance is negative during tests of concentrating ability and is decreased when less plasma filtrate passes through the glomerular membrane, when there is excessive secretion of antidiuretic hormone, and in patients with heart failure and liver damage. Free water clearance is increased in tests of diluting ability and is elevated in patients with diabetes insipidus, adrenal insufficiency, and certain head injuries.

DETERMINATIONS

Osmotic pressure is measured indirectly by determining depression of either the freezing point or the vapor pressure of the urine. The differences between the freezing points and vapor pressures of water and of an aqueous solution (in this instance, urine) are directly proportional to the molality of the solutions. A one molal solution, 1000 mOsm/kg, depresses the freezing point 1.86° C below the 0° C freezing point of water.

Osmolality can be determined on as little as 3 ml of urine by measuring freezing point depression with a freezing point osmometer (Fig. 11). These instruments are calibrated for both temperature and osmolality readings.

Until recently, freezing point depression was the only practical method of determining osmolality. A vapor pressure osmometer is now available also. It is relatively simple and easy to use and requires only a few drops of urine for the determination. An advantage of this method is that osmolality can now be measured at any selected temperature.

OSMOMETER

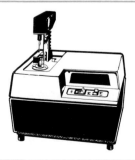

Figure 11.

URINE pH

7.

The kidneys and the lungs are the two major organs that regulate the acid-base balance of the body. The lungs excrete carbon dioxide while the kidneys regulate the excretion of the nonvolatile acids produced by the normal metabolic processes of the tissues. The acidity of urine is due primarily to acid phosphates, with only a minor portion contributed by organic acids such as pyruvic, lactic, and citric acids. These acids are excreted in the urine as salts, primarily sodium, potassium, calcium, and ammonium salts. The kidney regulates the selective excretion of the various cations in order to maintain normal acid-base balance. This is accomplished primarily through the reabsorption of a variable amount of sodium ion by the tubules and the concomitant tubular secretion of hydrogen and ammonium ions in exchange. Urine becomes increasingly acid as the amount of sodium retained by the body increases.

REFERENCE VALUES

The pH of the urine is a measure of the hydrogen ion concentration of the urine (Figure 12). A pH below 7 indicates acid urine; a pH above 7, alkaline urine. Normal kidneys are capable of producing urine that can vary from a pH of 4.5 to slightly higher than 8.0. Freshly voided urine from patients on normal diets is acid and has a pH of about 6.0. Normal blood pH ranges from 7.34 to 7.42.

ACID URINE

Acid urine, with pH lower than 6.0, may be excreted by patients on high protein diets. Certain medications such as ammonium chloride and mandelic acid may also produce acid urines. Patients with acidosis and/or uncontrolled diabetes mellitus excrete urine containing large amounts of acid.

ALKALINE URINE

Alkaline urine is frequently excreted after meals as a normal response to the secretion of HCl in the gastric juice. It also occurs in individuals consuming diets high in vegetables, milk and other dairy products. Certain medicines, such as sodium bicarbonate, potassium citrate, and acetazolamide, induce the formation of alkaline urine. Renal tubular acidosis is a specific disease of the kidneys in which the renal tubules are unable to adequately excrete hydrogen ions although severe systemic acidosis is present within the body. The urine pH of these patients usually remains approximately neutral and never falls below pH 5.0. A similar defect in hydrogen ion excretion occurs in the Fanconi syndrome. Highly alkaline urines may represent either urinary tract infection or possible bacterial contamination of the specimen with urea splitting organisms.

Certain antibiotics (such as neomycin, kanamycin, and streptomycin) are most effective in the treatment of urinary tract infections when they are excreted in alkaline urine. Salicylate excretion is enhanced by alkalinity. Renal stone formation partially depends on the pH of urine. Phosphate and calcium carbonate calculi develop in alkaline urine while uric acid, cystine, and calcium oxalate stones precipitate in acid urine.

ACID/ALKALINE URINE

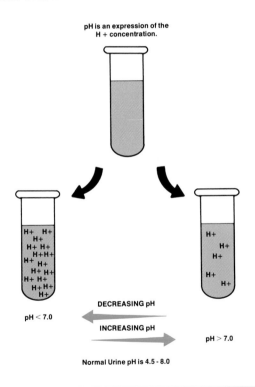

pH is an expression of the H + concentration.

DECREASING pH

pH < 7.0

INCREASING pH

pH > 7.0

Normal Urine pH is 4.5 - 8.0

Figure 12.

DETERMINATIONS

The accurate measurement of urinary pH can be done only on freshly voided specimens. Urine may become alkaline upon standing because of the loss of carbon dioxide and the conversion of urea into ammonia by certain bacterial organisms. If urine must be kept for any prolonged length of time before analysis, it should be stored in a container of approximately the same volume and refrigerated.

For routine analysis, urinary pH may be measured with indicator paper strips and a color chart. When more exact determinations are needed, a pH meter is used and the answer obtained directly from the meter.

A variety of test papers impregnated with various chemicals are available for the easy and rapid colorimetric determination of pH. Since urine pH is almost always measured as part of the more complete urinalysis, it is advantageous to use a multiple determination reagent strip such as COMBISTIX® Reagent Strip, HEMA-COMBISTIX® Reagent Strip, LABSTIX® Reagent Strip, BILI-LABSTIX® Reagent Strip, MULTISTIX® Reagent Strip, N-MULTISTIX® Reagent Strip, or N-MULTISTIX® SG Reagent Strip that simultaneously measures pH and checks the urine for several other components.

The pH portion of each of these strips is impregnated with two separate indicators, methyl red and bromthymol blue. These chemicals provide a wide spectrum of color changes, from orange to green to blue, in the pH range of 5 to 8.5. The reagent strip is dipped into the urine specimen and the color change is compared to a standardized color chart on the bottle label which shows pH values 5 through 8.5 in steps of 0.5 pH unit.

Nitrazine indicator papers are sensitive and specific in the pH range of 4.0 to 8.0. Several wide-range pH papers are also available but are not particularly useful for determinations of urinary pH because the increments on the color scale are too great for close pH approximations.

URINE VOLUME

8.

The normal volume of urine voided by an adult in a 24-hour period ranges from 750 to 2000 ml; the average volume is about 1500 ml. The amount voided over any period is directly related to the individual's fluid intake, the temperature and climate, and the amount of perspiration that occurs. Children void somewhat smaller quantities than adults do, but the total volume voided is greater in proportion to their body size.

POLYURIA

Polyuria is the increased excretion of urine. It is a physiologic response to increased fluid intake; the ingestion of diuretic medications; certain diuretic drinks, such as coffee, tea, and alcohol; chilling of the body; nervousness and anxiety; and the intravenous infusion of fluids.

Polyuria occurs in several disease states, particularly in diabetes mellitus and diabetes insipidus. It is a symptom of chronic renal disease, and it has been noted in patients with certain tumors of the brain and spinal cord, acromegaly, and myxedema. Polyuria may indicate the loss of concentrating ability by the kidneys.

OLIGURIA AND ANURIA

Oliguria is decreased urinary output (i.e., less than 200 ml/24-hours), the extreme form of which is anuria, a total lack of urine. Physiologic forms of oliguria occur with decreased fluid intake, increased ingestion of salt, and excessive perspiration.

Oliguria occurs when there is excessive loss of body fluid as in vomiting and diarrhea; when there is renal shutdown either through inflammation (nephritis), poisoning, or in cardiac insufficiency. Occasionally oliguria occurs due to mechanical obstruction to the urinary flow.

Measurement of urine volume is performed by pouring the timed specimen sample into a large graduated cylinder and recording the volume in milliliters. The total volume recorded is reported as urine volume per unit of time (generally 24 hours).

PROTEINS IN URINE

9.

REFERENCE VALUES

Normally an amount of protein between 40 and 80 mg is excreted per day, but as much as 100 to 150 mg per day may be considered within normal limits. Since the average daily urine volume may range from 1000 to 1500 ml, the average normal concentration of protein in the urine varies from 2 to 8 mg/dL. This wide range in the so called normal values is the result of biological variations and differences in methods used for the determination of protein.

Approximately one-third of normal urinary protein is albumin. This albumin appears to be identical to serum albumin. The majority of normal proteins in the urine are globulins. These globulins primarily consist of alpha-1 and alpha-2 globulins, with smaller amounts of beta and gamma globulins. Urine globulins have lower molecular weight than the corresponding serum globulins but are antigenically closely related. Trace quantities of other proteins may also be found in most urine. A high molecular weight mucoprotein, the Tamm-Horsfall protein, occurs in normal urine in quantities up to 2.5 mg/dL. In nephrosis it may occur in higher concentrations. It is not found in plasma and is thought to originate in the kidney.

CLINICAL UTILITY

Proteinuria refers to an increased amount of protein in the urine. Proteinuria is probably one of the single most important indicators of renal disease. Detection of protein in the urine combined with the microscopic examination of the urinary sediment forms the basis of the differential laboratory diagnosis of renal disorders. Proteinuria may, at times, reflect extrarenal disease rather than intrinsic renal disorders.

The type of protein excreted in disease states is generally related to the serum proteins; in fact, in severe cases, they are the serum proteins. Smaller proteins, such as albumin and alpha-1 globulin, are excreted more readily than larger ones. Albumin constitutes between 60 and 90 percent of protein excreted in most disease states. Certain diseases are characterized by the excretion of specific globulins rather than by a diffuse proteinuria. The urine of patients with multiple myeloma contains increased amounts of a low molecular weight globulin (Bence Jones protein). Bence Jones proteinuria may also be found in some patients with macroglobinemia and primary systemic amyloidosis. An increased excretion of a specific globulin that is similar to Bence Jones protein occurs in Franklin's disease, and patients with renal tubular disorders, such as the Fanconi syndrome, show a predominant increase in the quantities of globulins excreted in the urine. (Table 2)

Proteinuria depends upon the precise nature of the clinical and pathological disorder and upon the severity of the specific disease. Proteinuria may be intermittent or continuous; transient, intermittent proteinuria is usually caused by physiologic or functional conditions rather than by renal disorders.

Marked proteinuria is characterized by the excretion of more than 4 gm per day. It is typical of the nephrotic syndrome but also occurs in severe cases of glomerulonephritis, nephrosclerosis, amyloid disease, systemic lupus erythematosus, and severe venous congestion of the kidney produced by renal vein thrombosis, congestive heart failure, or constrictive pericarditis.

Moderate proteinuria refers to the daily excretion of between 0.5 and 4 gm. of protein. It is found in the vast majority of renal diseases, all of the disorders listed above, chronic glomerulonephritis, diabetic nephropathy, multiple myeloma, toxic nephropathy, preeclampsia, and inflammatory, malignant, degenerative, and irritative conditions of the lower urinary tract, including the presence of calculi.

Minimal proteinuria is the excretion of less than 0.5 gm of protein per day. It is associated with chronic glomerulonephritis, polycystic disease of the kidneys, renal tubular disorders, the healing phase of acute glomerulonephritis, latent or inactive stages of glomerulonephritis, and various disorders of the lower urinary tract.

Postural proteinuria is excretion of protein by patients who are erect or in the lordotic position. The proteinuria is intermittent and disappears when the individual lies down. The daily protein excretion usually is less than 1 gm. Postural proteinuria occurs in three to five percent of healthy young adults. It may be differentiated from other forms of proteinuria by testing for protein in urine specimens collected before and after the individual has been erect. The patient voids and discards his urine at bedtime. He collects a urine specimen immediately after awakening and before he is upright for more than a moment. He collects another specimen after he has remained erect or walking for a period of at least two hours. The first specimen should contain no protein. The second will be positive if the patient has postural proteinuria.

Functional proteinuria is protein excretion in association with fever, exposure to heat or cold, excessive exercise, and emotional stress. The underlying physiologic mechanism that induces proteinuria in all of these is renal vasoconstriction.

Table 2

PROTEINS IN URINE

PROTEIN	CONDITION(S)
Albumin	Strenuous Physical Exercise Emotional Stress Pregnancy Infections Glomerulonephritis Newborns (1st week)
Globulins	Glomerulonephritis Tubular Dysfunction
Hemoglobin	Hematuria Hemoglobinuria
Fibrinogen	Severe Renal Disease
Nucleoproteins	WBC's in urine Epithelial cells in urine
Bence-Jones	Multiple myeloma Leukemia

Bence Jones protein is a specific low molecular weight protein excreted in the urine of more than half of patients with multiple myeloma. It is also found in the urine of many patients with macroglobulinemia. This protein represents a portion of the high molecular weight plasma myeloma globulin. It is different from all other urinary proteins in that it coagulates on heating to temperatures between 45° to 60° C and then redissolves on further heating to the boiling point.

DETERMINATIONS

A number of simple, semiquantitative tests and more complex quantitative tests are available for the determination of all proteins in urine. Specific methods are used for the detection and quantitation of albumin, globulins, Bence Jones protein and others. The majority of these methods, with the notable exception of the simple colorimetric reagent strip test, depend upon the precipitation of protein as the basis for quantitative determinations. Table 3 shows a clinical approach to proteinuria.

Table 3 **PROTEINURIA: CLINICAL APPROACH**

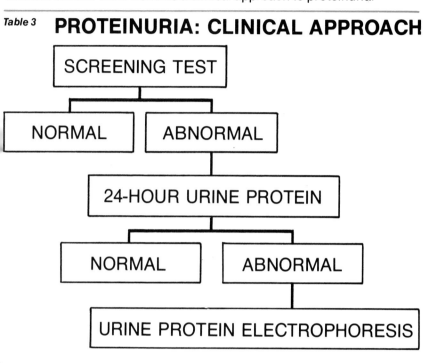

COLORIMETRIC REAGENT STRIP TEST

The colorimetric reagent strip test is based upon the ability of proteins to alter the color of some acid-base indicators without altering the pH. When an indicator such as tetrabromphenol blue is buffered at pH 3, it is yellow in solutions without protein, but in the presence of protein the color will change to green and then to blue with increasing protein concentrations.

ALBUSTIX® Reagent Strip is a protein test strip that contains a single test area. This area consists of a small square of absorbent paper impregnated with a buffered solution of tetrabromphenol blue. URISTIX®, N-URISTIX™, COMBISTIX®, HEMA-COMBISTIX®, LABSTIX®, BILI-LABSTIX®, MULTISTIX® and N-MULTISTIX® and N-MULTISTIX®-SG Reagent Strips are multi-determinant reagent strips, each containing an area for protein determination along with test areas for other urinary constituents. Protein is determined simply by dipping the strip into well-mixed uncentrifuged urine, and immediately comparing the resultant color with the chart provided on the reagent strip bottle. The results are reported as negative (yellow color), trace, or one "plus" to four "plus". Trace readings may detect 5 to 20 mg of protein/dL.

"Plus" readings are approximately equivalent to protein concentrations of 30, 100, 300, and over 2000/dL respectively and are reliable indicators of increasingly severe proteinuria. Albumin reacts with the indicator more strongly than do the other proteins. Highly buffered, alkaline urines may give false positives when the buffer systems in the reagent area is overcome and an actual shift in pH of the buffers occurs.

SEMIQUANTITATIVE PRECIPITATION TESTS

The heat and acetic acid method, the sulfosalicylic acid method, and the concentrated nitric acid protein precipitation method are three simple methods for semiquantitating protein concentration in terms of trace through four plus precipitation. The precipitation is read and interpreted as follows:

Negative means no turbidity.
Trace is a faint precipitate visible against a black background, equivalent to about 5 mg/dL protein.
One plus is a small degree of turbidity, equivalent to 10 to 30 mg/dL.
Two plus is a moderate turbidity equivalent to 40 to 100 mg/dL.
Three plus is heavy turbidity equivalent to 200 to 500 mg/dL.
Four plus is heavy flocculation equivalent to 500 mg/dL or more.

＊

Heat and acetic acid technique
1. Place 5 to 10 ml clear urine in a test tube. If urine is not clear, centrifuge or filter first.
2. Boil the upper portion over a flame.
3. If turbidity develops, add 1 to 3 drops of glacial acetic acid. Any turbidity due to phosphate precipitation will clear.
4. Reboil and estimate the amount of turbidity as an index of the amount of protein present.

This method is the most sensitive for small amounts of protein and can reliably detect protein concentrations of 2 to 3mg/dL.

Sulfosalicylic acid method
1. Place 4 to 5 ml urine in a test tube.
2. Add 2 to 3 drops of 20% sulfosalicylic acid.
3. Mix thoroughly and estimate the amount of turbidity.
An alternate method is to use BUMINTEST® tablets.
1. Prepare reagent solution by dissolving 4 BUMINTEST® tablets in 30 ml of water.

2. Place 10 drops of the solution and 10 drops of urine in a test tube.
3. Shake tube gently and observe for turbidity.

Nitric acid test
1. Place 2 to 3 ml of concentrated nitric acid in a test tube.
2. Carefully pour about 5 ml of clear urine (filter first if necessary) down the inner side of the inclined test tube so that the urine forms a layer over the nitric acid.
3. A ring of precipitated protein will form at the interface. Estimate the amount of precipitate.

QUANTITATIVE 24 HOUR PROTEIN DETERMINATIONS

Simple estimates of the protein content of urine are performed by quantitating the amount of precipitation formed following the addition of a specific chemical to the urine. The precipitate is measured either by comparison with known standards or by recording the height of the column of precipitate in a specially devised tube. More complex quantitative tests involve the measurement of protein precipitation with a nephelometer or photometer. These tests usually are adaptations of one of the other precipitation tests such as the sulfosalicylic acid turbidity test.

Sulfosalicylic acid turbidity test
1. Pipette 2.5 ml of centrifuged urine into a test tube.
2. Add 7.5 ml of 3% sulfosalicylic acid. (3 gm diluted with water to 100 ml).
3. Invert to mix.
4. Let stand 10 minutes.
5. Compare the turbidity with known standards prepared from solutions containing 10, 20, 30 ,40, 50, 75, and 100 mg albumin/dL, and estimate the concentration of the unknown. If the unknown urine contains more than 100 mg/dL protein, dilute the urine and repeat the test.

BENCE JONES PROTEIN DETERMINATION

Bence Jones protein is soluble at room and body temperatures. It precipitates upon heating between 45° and 60° C, and then redissolves when the urine is further heated to the boiling point.

Gradual heating of a urine sample to the boiling point is the simplest screening method for Bence Jones protein. When present, a precipitate will first appear and then redissolve as the urine is further heated. The presence of large amounts of other proteins or phosphates decreases the accuracy of this test. These interfering proteins can usually be removed by cooling the heated urine to room temperature, filtering and repeating the heating process on the filtrate.

Acetic acid test
1. Place 4.0 ml clear urine in a test tube (centrifuge if necessary).

2. Add 1.0 ml acetate buffer (add 17.5 gm sodium acetate trihydrate and 4.1 ml glacial acetic acid to distilled water; dilute to 100 ml with distilled water).
3. Place in a 56° C water bath and heat for 15 minutes.
4. Precipitation indicates the presence of Bence Jones proteinuria.
5. If precipitation occurs, heat the tube in boiling water for 3 minutes and observe. Bence Jones protein will redissolve.
6. Cool tube. Precipitation will recur as solution cools to 45-60° C and redissolve as the solution cools below 40° C.

SUGAR IN URINE

10.

GLUCOSE

Glucose is the sugar most commonly found in urine; although other sugars such as lactose, fructose, galactose, and pentose may also be found under certain conditions.

The presence of detectable amounts of glucose in urine is known as *glucosuria* or *glycosuria* (either is correct). Glucosuria occurs whenever the blood glucose level exceeds the reabsorption capacity of the renal tubules, i.e., when the glomerular filtrate contains more glucose than the tubules are able to reabsorb (renal threshold). The condition may be either benign or pathological, and the physician must distinguish between the two types.

Renal glucosuria occurs with normal blood glucose levels because tubular reabsorption of glucose is below normal, thus permitting some glucose to spill into the urine. This is a benign condition as is the occurrence of glucosuria after eating a heavy meal or in conjunction with emotional stress.

Diabetes mellitus, a pathological state, is the chief cause of glucosuria. This condition is associated with a marked elevation of blood sugar levels and usually an increase in urine volume. The sugar content of a diabetic urine may reach as high as 10%, but 2-5% values are more commonly found. The urine is usually light in color with increased specific gravity due to the extra load of dissolved solids.

DETERMINATIONS

There are a variety of tests for glucose which may be applied to urine. Those most frequently used are of two types: (1) reduction tests based upon the reduction of certain metal ions by glucose, and (2) enzymatic tests based upon the action of glucose oxidase upon glucose. Table 4 gives the chemical principle of selected glucose tests.

Table 4 **CHEMICAL PRINCIPLE OF SELECTED GLUCOSE TESTS**

■ **Copper Reduction—CLINITEST®, Benedict's**

Cupric ions ($CuSO_4$) **Blue**	+ Glucose (or reducing substance)	heat $\rightarrow$ alkali	Cuprous ions (Cu_2O) **Orange-red**	+	Oxidized Glucose

Table 4 (cont'd)

■ **Enzymatic—CLINISTIX®**

$$\text{Glucose} + O_2 \,(\text{air}) \xrightarrow[\text{oxidase}]{\text{glucose}} \begin{array}{c} \text{Gluconic} \\ \text{Acid} \end{array} + \begin{array}{c} \text{Hydrogen} \\ \text{Peroxide} \end{array}$$

$$\begin{array}{c} \text{Hydrogen} \\ \text{Peroxide} \end{array} + \begin{array}{c} \text{Chromogen} \\ \text{(o-tolidine)} \end{array} \xrightarrow[\rightarrow]{\text{peroxidase}} \begin{array}{c} \text{Oxidized} \\ \text{O-tolidine} \\ \textbf{Blue} \end{array} + H_2O$$

■ **Enzymatic—DIASTIX®, KETO-DIASTIX®, AMES' MULTIPLES**

$$\text{Glucose} + O_2 \,(\text{air}) \xrightarrow[\text{oxidase}]{\text{glucose}} \begin{array}{c} \text{Gluconic} \\ \text{Acid} \end{array} + \begin{array}{c} \text{Hydrogen} \\ \text{Peroxide} \end{array}$$

$$\begin{array}{c} \text{Hydrogen} \\ \text{Peroxide} \end{array} + \begin{array}{c} \text{Chromogen} \\ \text{(Iodine} \\ \text{Complex)} \end{array} \xrightarrow[\rightarrow]{\text{peroxidase}} \begin{array}{c} \text{Oxidized} \\ \text{Iodine} \\ \text{Complex} \\ \textbf{Brown} \end{array} + H_2O$$

REDUCTION TESTS

The reduction of metallic ions such as Cu^{++} is nonspecific for glucose since the reaction may be brought about by any reducing substance that may be present in the urine, such as creatinine, uric acid, ascorbic acid, or some other reducing sugar. Noncarbohydrate components seldom interfere, but occasionally in concentrated urines, some interference may occur. The nonspecificity of the copper reduction tests can be both an advantage in that they will detect sugar other than glucose, and a disadvantage in that false positives may also occur. (Table 4)

Benedict's Test

Benedict's reagent consists of copper sulfate dissolved in a sodium carbonate, sodium citrate solution. It is used by placing 5 ml. in a test tube, adding 5 to 8 drops of urine, and placing the tube in a boiling water bath for five minutes. After heating, the tube is removed from the bath, allowed to cool in the air, and the color noted. The color varies from blue (no reducing substance or sugar present), through green, to yellow, to orange, to a brick red color indicating a sugar or some other reducing substance is present. The amount of reducing substance present can be roughly estimated by noting the degree of color change as compared to test urines containing a known amount of glucose. As little as 0.1% (100 mg/dL) glucose is capable of giving a positive reaction with Benedict's reagent.

CLINITEST® REAGENT TABLET

The copper reduction test has been greatly simplified by CLINITEST®, which consists of copper sulfate compounded into an effervescent tablet containing sodium carbonate, citric acid, and sodium hydroxide. When the tablet is added to a small test tube containing 10 drops of water and 5 drops of urine (5-drop method), it dissolves with the evolution of carbon dioxide and heat. In the process, if a reducing substance such as glucose is present, the color changes from blue to orange, depending upon the amount of sugar present. By comparing the color with a reference color chart, the amount of reducing substance in the urine can be estimated. The 2-drop method is the same as above, except that 2 drops of urine is used and the results are compared to a special 2-drop color chart.

CLINITEST® is sensitive to approximately 0.25% glucose in urine. It is somewhat less sensitive than Benedict's reagent, but on the other hand, it gives fewer false positive reactions.

Nylander's Test

Nylander's test is based upon the reduction of alkaline bismuth subnitrate by glucose. When heated, a mixture of Nylander's reagent and urine containing glucose will produce a black precipitate of free bismuth.

ENZYMATIC TESTS

The enzymatic methods as they are applied to urine are specific for glucose, although some components such as ascorbic acid may inhibit the test. (Table 4)

GLUCOSE OXIDASE TESTS

The enzymatic glucose oxidase tests for glucose, as applied to urine, are specific for glucose. In these tests, glucose oxidase catalyzes the oxidation of glucose to gluconolactone and a peroxide. The peroxide in the presence of peroxidase is used to oxidize an indicator which in turn produces a color change. Sugars such as lactose, fructose, galactose, and pentose are not substrates for glucose oxidase and therefore do not react with this test.

DIASTIX® Reagent Strips and the glucose test portions of URISTIX®, N-URISTIX®, COMBISTIX®, HEMA-COMBISTIX®, LABSTIX®, BILI-LABSTIX®, MULTISTIX® and N-MULTISTIX®, N-MULTISTIX®-SG contain a glucose oxidase test system and are specific for glucose.

In practice, the test strips are dipped into the urine sample, the excess removed by touching the side of the container and the resulting glucose color reaction is compared to a six-block color chart ranging from blue, indicating less than 0.1% concentration of glucose, to brown at 2.0% or more. The DIASTIX® test is read at 30 seconds.

CLINISTIX® Reagent Strip is another glucose test strip using the glucose oxidase principle. The results of this test are primarily qualitative. Quantitation is only approximate because of the variable effect different urines may have on the color development. Lily's Tes-Tape® is based on the same principle. If quantitation is desired, CLINITEST® or DIASTIX® should be used. CLINITEST® will detect any sugar present in urine; whereas the glucose test strips, DIASTIX® and CLINISTIX®, will distinguish urines containing glucose only. It is important to remember that both DIASTIX® and CLINISTIX® are sensitive to glucose at the 0.1% (100 mg/dL) level; thus, they may give a positive reaction when CLINITEST® is negative since sensitivity of the latter is set at 0.25% (250 mg/dL).

NON-GLUCOSE REDUCING SUGARS

As CLINITEST® reacts with all reducing sugars, a positive result will be observed whenever such sugars, e.g., lactose, galactose, fructose, or pentose are present.

LACTOSE

Lactose may appear in the urine of lactating women. This is usually a temporary condition which corrects itself upon the cessation of lactation. It may be found in trace amounts of the urine of three to five-day old infants before their digestive systems have become fully developed, and in other children and adults who are deficient in intestinal lactase.

The presence of lactose in urine can be detected by CLINITEST®. Identifying the sugar as lactose, although not a routine procedure, can be done by the mucic acid test, the osazone test, paper chromatography, and hydrolyzing the sugar and testing for galactose by the galactose oxidase method. The presence of lactose in urine is usually considered physiological rather than pathological.

GALACTOSE

Galactose is found in the urine of infants afflicted with galactosemia. These children are deficient in the enzyme necessary for converting galactose into glucose. This is a severe condition which can be treated by eliminating lactose and other sources of galactose from the diet. If not done, the infants will rapidly deteriorate physically and mentally to an early demise. Occasionally, adults who ingest large quantities of milk or other lactose-containing foods will show trace amounts of galactose in the urine. This has no clinical significance and disappears upon the reduction of galactose intake.

Galactose can be detected with CLINITEST® and identified by the mucic acid test, osazone test, paper chromatography, and by the galactose oxidase test. Some pediatricians will screen infants urine with CLINITEST® and CLINISTIX® to detect the presence of a non-glucose reducing substance, i.e., positive CLINITEST®, negative CLINISTIX®.

FRUCTOSE

Fructose sometimes occurs in the urine of patients with hepatic disorders. Its presence can be detected with CLINITEST®. It can be identified by Selivanoff's test, and by paper chromatography, neither of which is a routine procedure.

PENTOSE

Pentosuria is associated with certain types of drug therapy and with some hereditary conditions. In both cases, its presence in urine is considered benign, but its presence can cause diagnostic problems. Its presence can be detected with CLINITEST®, and it will reduce Benedict's reagent at room temperature.

Identification of a pentose can be done by Tauber's test, osazone test, and paper chromatography.

KETONES IN URINE

11.

The body normally metabolizes fats completely to carbon dioxide and water. Whenever there is inadequate carbohydrate in the diet or a defect in carbohydrate metabolism or absorption: the body metabolizes increasing amounts of fatty acids. When this increase is large, fatty acid utilization is incomplete. Intermediary products of fat metabolism appear in the blood and are excreted in the urine. These intermediary products are the three ketone bodies: acetoacetic acid (which is also called diacetic acid), acetone, and betahydroxybutyric acid. Acetone and betahydroxybutyric acid are derived from acetoacetic acid. All three ketone bodies are present in the urine of patients with ketonuria in the relative proportions of 20% acetoacetic acid, 2% acetone, and 78% betahydroxybutyric acid. (Figure 13)

CLINICAL UTILITY—KETONURIA

Diabetes mellitus is the most important disorder in which ketonuria occurs. Diabetes mellitus is a disorder of glucose metabolism, and in insulin-deficient diabetes (usually the juvenile-onset type), glucose metabolism is sufficiently impaired that fatty acids are utilized to meet the body's energy requirements. When this type of diabetes is untreated or inadequately treated, excessive amounts of fatty acids are metabolized, with the result that ketone bodies accumulate in blood (ketosis) and are excreted in urine (ketonuria). Ketone bodies are excreted in combination with normal basic ions, leading to a reduction in the carbon dioxide combining power and causing systemic acidosis. Progressive diabetic ketosis is the cause of diabetic acidosis which can eventually lead to coma and even death. The term ketoacidosis is frequently used to designate the combined ketosis and acidosis of diabetes.

Thus, detection of ketonuria in a patient with diabetes mellitus is of great significance since a change in insulin dosage or other management procedures is often indicated. During periods of acute infections, surgery, gastrointestinal disturbances, or other stress, and whenever the management routine does not adequately control the disease, the urine of all diabetic patients should be checked for the presence of ketone bodies.

Ketonuria also accompanies the restricted carbohydrate intake that occurs in association with fevers, anorexia, gastrointestinal disturbances, fasting, starvation, cyclic vomiting, pernicious vomiting of pregnancy, cachexia, following anesthesia, and as a result of certain neurologic disorders. One popular diet which restricted carbohydrates called for monitoring progress of the diet by measuring ketones in the urine.

**FATTY ACID METABOLISM WITH
IMPAIRED GLUCOSE OXIDATION**

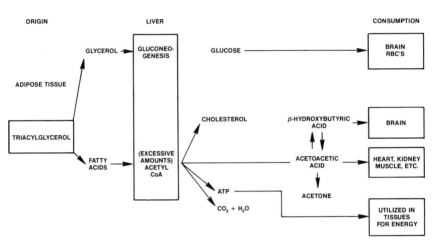

Figure 13

DETERMINATIONS

In ketonuria acetoacetic acid, acetone, and betahydroxybutyric acid are all excreted in the urine. Consequently, a test procedure which principally determines one of these three components is generally satisfactory for the diagnosis of ketonuria. Specific tests do exist for the determination of each of these substances but they are not generally used because the methods are more cumbersome and they are less reliable and less sensitive.

Nitroprusside reactions:

Nitroprusside generally reacts with both acetone and acetoacetic acid in the presence of alkali to produce a purple-colored compound. This forms the basis of a number of different tests.

The *reagent strip method* is the simplest technique for determination of ketonuria. The KETOSTIX® Reagent Strip, is impregnated with sodium nitroprusside buffers. The strip is dipped into fresh urine, tapped to remove excess urine, and compared to the color chart after exactly 15 seconds. The chart has six color blocks, indicating negative, trace, small, moderate, large 80 and large 160 concentrations of ketones, and ranging in color from buff to lavender and maroon. The test is sensitive to aceto-

49

acetic acid. It does not react with betahydroxybutyric acid or acetone. KETO-DIASTIX®, LABSTIX®, BILI-LABSTIX®, MULTISTIX®, N-MULTISTIX® and N-MULTISTIX®-SG reagent strips also contain reagent areas for detecting acetoacetic acid.

Rothera's Test

1. Add about 1 gm Rothera's reagent to 5 ml of urine in a test tube.
2. Layer over the urine 1 to 2 ml concentrated ammonium hydroxide by allowing it to flow gently down the side of the inclined test tube.
3. When ketones are present, a pink-purple ring develops at the interface. The results range from a 1+ pink reaction to a 4+ dark purple red reaction. A negative result shows no ring or a brown ring.

Rothera's reagent:

sodium nitroprusside	7.5 gm
ammonium sulfate	200.0 gm

Mix and pulverize.

This test has been largely replaced by the use of reagent strips.

Legal's Test

1. Place 3 to 4 ml urine in a test tube.
2. Add enough sodium or potassium hydroxide solution to make the urine alkaline.
3. Add a few drops of sodium nitroprusside solution, made by dissolving a few crystals of sodium nitroprusside in 2 ml distilled water.
4. Add a few drops of concentrated acetic acid.
5. In the presence of acetone or acetoacetic acid, the solution turns red to purple. This test also has generally been replaced by the use of reagent strips.

Ferric chloride test for acetoacetic acid—Gerhardt's Test

1. Place 5 ml urine in a test tube.
2. Add 10% ferric chloride solution (10 gm ferric chloride in 100 ml distilled water) drop by drop, agitating well, until the precipitate that develops has redissolved.
3. If acetoacetic acid is present, the solution turns a deep red color.
4. Many other substances, including salicylates, give positive color reactions. To differentiate acetoacetic acid from them, the urine must be boiled for 15 minutes. This converts acetoacetic acid to acetone and a positive result will no longer be obtained.

Hart's Test—betahydroxybutyric acid

1. Place 20 ml urine in a beaker.
2. Add 20 ml distilled water and a few drops of acetic acid.

3. Boil until the volume is reduced to 10 ml. This removes acetone and acetoacetic acid.
4. Dilute to 20 ml with distilled water and divide into two equal portions.
5. Add 1 ml hydrogen peroxide to one portion. Heat gently, then let cool.
6. Test both portions for acetone with the Legal nitroprusside method.
7. When betahydroxybutyric acid is present, the tube containing the hydrogen peroxide will show a red ring at the interface.

ACETEST® Reagent Tablet—
Detection of acetone and acetoacetic acid
1. Place tablet on a clean surface, preferably a piece of white paper.
2. Put one drop of urine (serum, plasma, or whole blood) on tablet.
3. Compare urine ketone test results to color chart at 30 seconds.* (Make serum or plasma ketone readings 2 minutes after application of specimen to tablet. When testing for ketones in whole blood, wait 10 minutes before removing clotted blood from tablet and read results immediately.)

---

*To test the absorptive quality of the tablet, place a drop of urine on tablet. The drop of urine should be completely absorbed into the tablet within a 30-second period. If absorption of the urine into the tablet takes longer than 30 seconds, the tablet has been exposed to moisture and may give a faulty reading.

HEMOGLOBIN AND RED BLOOD CELLS IN URINE

12.

Hemoglobin is the oxygen-carrying pigment of red blood cells. When hemolysis (lysis of red blood cells) occurs, free hemoglobin is released into the surrounding medium. If hemolysis occurs in the circulation (for example, in hemolytic anemia), free hemoglobin is present in the blood; when present in sufficient quantity, significant amounts enter the glomerular filtrate and appear in the urine. When red blood cells enter the urine at any point in the urinary tract (as a result of disease or trauma), hemolysis may occur in the urine, with the release of detectable amounts of free hemoglobin.

CLINICAL UTILITY

The hemolysis that produces hemoglobinuria may have occurred in the bloodstream, in a particular body organ, in the kidney or lower urinary tract, or in the urine sample itself. Hemoglobinuria may indicate a hematologic disorder such as hemolytic anemia, hemolytic transfusion reaction, paroxysmal nocturnal hemoglobinuria, paroxysmal cold hemoglobinuria, or favism (a glucose-6-phosphate dehydrogenase deficiency). Hemoglobinuria is found in severe infectious diseases such as yellow fever, smallpox, and malaria; in poisonings with strong acids or mushrooms; following burns; and with renal infarction. A significant amount of free hemoglobin is found in the urine whenever red blood cells are present in excessive numbers as a result of frank or occult bleeding that may accompany various renal disorders, or infectious or neoplastic disease or trauma affecting any part of the urinary tract.

DETERMINATIONS

The reagent strip test is the simplest and most direct test for the presence of hemoglobin in urine. The reagent area is impregnated with tetramethylbenzidine and buffered organic peroxide. Tetramethylbenzidine forms a green to dark blue compound when hemoglobin catalyzes the oxidation reaction of tetramethylbenzidine with a peroxide. Development of green spots indicate non-hemolyzed (intact) erythrocytes.

The color of the strip is compared with a color chart 40 seconds after the strip is dipped into the urine. The color blocks indicate negative, non-hemolyzed trace, hemolyzed trace, small (+), moderate (++) and large amounts (+++) of hemoglobin and range in color from orange through green to blue. Myoglobin, if present in large enough concentrations, will give a positive reaction. The AMES Company multiple urine strips from HEMA-COMBISTIX® up contain test areas with the same chemical reagents for the determination of hemoglobin. The test is generally capable of detecting 0.015 to 0.060 mg/dL free hemoglobin or 5 to 20 intact red blood cells per microliter. Large amounts of ascorbic acid (Vitamin C) in the urine may inhibit or retard the reaction.

BILIRUBIN IN URINE

13.

Bilirubin in the urine indicates the presence of hepatocellular disease or intra- or extrahepatic biliary obstruction. It is an early sign of these disorders and, therefore, a useful diagnostic tool. Bilirubin is formed in the reticuloendothelial cells of the spleen and bone marrow from the breakdown of hemoglobin. It is linked to albumin in the bloodstream and transported to the liver. This albumin-bound form, which is also known as indirect bilirubin, is insoluble in water and does not appear in the urine except in trace amounts. In the liver cells, it is separated from the albumin and conjugated with glucuronic and sulfuric acids to form water-soluble conjugated bilirubin, also known as direct bilirubin. The liver cells that form the conjugated bilirubin secrete it into the bile and thus it is excreted into the intestinal tract through the bile duct. This conjugated bilirubin in the intestinal tract is converted by bacterial action to urobilinogen. Being water-soluble, conjugated bilirubin can be excreted by the kidneys although normally its level in the blood is not sufficiently high to cause significant amounts to appear in the urine.

REFERENCE VALUES

Bilirubin present in urine is approximately 0.02 mg/dL, reflecting the normally low blood levels of conjugated bilirubin. This amount is undetected by routine semiquantitative techniques, and is interpreted as a negative result.

CLINICAL UTILITY

Bilirubin excretion in the urine will reach significant levels in any disease process that increases the amount of conjugated bilirubin in the bloodstream. In some liver diseases due to infectious or hepatotoxic agents, liver cells are unable to secrete all of the conjugated bilirubin in the bile, so that sufficient amounts are returned to the blood to elevate blood levels and cause significant bilirubinuria.

In obstructive biliary tract disease, biliary stasis interferes with the normal excretion of conjugated bilirubin via the intestinal tract, thus causing a build-up in the bloodstream with resulting bilirubinuria. Since bilirubin may often appear in the urine before other signs of liver dysfunction (jaundice, clinical illness) are apparent, bilirubinuria is an important diagnostic sign of liver disease and a bilirubin test should be part of every routine urinalysis.

Bilirubin excretion in the urine is not increased when there is an increase in the amount of unconjugated bilirubin in the circulation. This type of increase occurs in hemolytic anemias because the greater release of hemoglobin leads to greater production of albumin-bound bilirubin. However, a normal, non-diseased liver can conjugate all the excess bilirubin and secrete the entire amount into the biliary tract.

DETERMINATIONS

The bilirubin *reagent area* on BILI-LABSTIX® and higher multiple strips is the simplest semiquantitative test for the determination of bilirubin. The reagent area is impregnated with stabilized, diazotized 2, 4-dichloroaniline which reacts with bilirubin in urine to form a brownish to purplish colored azobilirubin compound. The reagent strip is dipped into fresh, uncentrifuged urine, tapped to remove excess urine, and after a 20-second wait, compared to the color chart on the reagent strip bottle. The results are interpreted as negative, or small, (+), moderate (+ +), and large amounts (+ + +) of bilirubin . The test has a sensitivity of 0.2 to 0.4 mg bilirubin/dL (Golden and Snavely procedure).

ICTOTEST® Reagent Tablets and special test mats are a highly sensitive and convenient method for the qualitative determination of bilirubinuria. ICTOTEST® Reagent Tablets contain P-nitrobenzenediazonium, P-toluenesulfonate, sodium bicarbonate, sulfosalicylic acid, and boric acid. The mats are made of an asbestos cellulose mixture.

1. Place 5 drops of urine on one special test mat; if bilirubin is present in the specimen, it will be absorbed onto the mat surface.
2. Place an ICTOTEST® Reagent Tablet on the moistened area of the mat.
3. Flow 2 drops of water on the tablet.
4. When elevated amounts of bilirubin are present in the urine specimen, a blue to purple color forms within 30 seconds. The rapidity of the formation of the color and the intensity of the color development are proportional to the amount of bilirubin in urine. Normal amounts of bilirubin in urine give a negative test result. The smallest concentration of bilirubin reliably detected by this method is 0.05 to 0.1 mg/dL. An orange to red color may indicate urobilin, indican, or salicylates in the urine.

Harrison Spot Test (Fouchet's Test)
1. Place 10 ml acidified urine in a test tube.
2. Add 5 ml 10% barium chloride solution.
3. Shake and filter.

4. To the residual precipitate on the filter paper, add 1 drop of reagent made as follows:

Trichloroacetic acid	25 gm
10% ferric chloride solution	10 ml
distilled water	100 ml

5. When bilirubin is present, a green or blue-green color develops.

Bilirubin is an unstable compound and disappears from urine on standing, especially if exposed to light. It is very important that urine be tested for bilirubin as soon after excretion as possible. (Figure 14)

BILIRUBIN IN URINE:

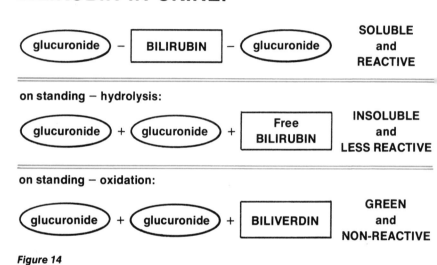

Figure 14

UROBILINOGEN IN URINE

14.

Conjugated bilirubin, secreted by the liver into the bile, is excreted into the intestinal tract through the bile duct. Bacterial action in the intestinal tract convert the bilirubin to a group of compounds known as urobilinogen. It is estimated that as much as 50% of the urobilinogen formed in the intestines is reabsorbed into the portal circulation and re-excreted by the liver. Small amounts are normally excreted in the urine, but the major excretion is in the feces.

REFERENCE VALUES

Normally between 1 and 4 mg of urobilinogen is excreted in urine in a 24 hour period. The concentration of urobilinogen in a random normal urine is 0.1 to 1.0 Ehrlich units/dL.

CLINICAL UTILITY

Urinary urobilinogen is increased by any condition that causes an increase in the production of bilirubin, and by any disease that prevents the liver from normally removing the reabsorbed urobilinogen from the portal circulation. Urinary urobilinogen is increased whenever there is excessive destruction of red blood cells as in hemolytic anemias, pernicious anemia, and malaria. It is increased also in infectious hepatitis, toxic hepatitis, portal cirrhosis, congestive heart failure, and infectious mononucleosis. Determinations of urinary urobilinogen are a useful procedure in routine urinalysis since they serve as a guide in detecting and differentiating liver disease, hemolytic disease, and biliary obstruction. Sequential determinations also assist in evaluating progress of the disease and response to management.

Urinary urobilinogen is decreased or absent when normal amounts of bilirubin are not excreted into the intestinal tract. This usually indicates partial or complete obstruction of the bile ducts such as may occur in cholelithiasis, severe inflammatory disease, or neoplastic disease. Also, during antibiotic therapy, suppression of normal intestinal flora may prevent conversion of bilirubin to urobilinogen, leading to absence of urobilinogen in urine.

More comprehensive information is obtained when the physician can correlate test results for both bilirubinuria and urobilinogenuria. As indicated in the correlation table below, the two findings, considered together, provide more helpful information for differential diagnosis than either finding alone, as shown below:

	In Health	In Hemolytic Disease	In Hepatic Disease	In Biliary Obstruction
Urine Urobilinogen	Normal	Increased	Increased	Low or Absence
Urine Bilirubin	Negative	Negative	Positive or Negative	Positive

DETERMINATIONS

UROBILISTIX® and a reagent area of MULTISTIX® and higher multiple Reagent Strips are impregnated with paradimethylaminobenzaldehyde, and an acid buffer solution. They react with urinary urobilinogen, porphobilinogen, and paraaminosalicylic acid, to form colored compounds. A freshly voided specimen of urine is necessary for the test, preferably a sample collected over a 2 hour period in the early afternoon when urinary urobilinogen excretion is thought to be at the highest rate for the day. The strip is dipped into fresh uncentrifuged urine collected without preservatives, removed and tapped free of excess urine. The color reaction is compared to the color chart after exactly 45 seconds.

The six color blocks provided on the chart range in color from light yellow to brown-orange, representing 0.1, 1, 2, 4, 6, and 12 Ehrlich units/100 dL of urine. The first two color blocks, 0.1 and 1 Ehrlich units/dL are within the normal range of values for urobilinogen. The remaining four color blocks indicate high values. This test will not accurately detect a decrease or absence of urobilinogen. No substances are known to clearly inhibit the reaction, but strongly alkaline urines will show higher urine urobilinogen values, and strongly acid urines show lower urobilinogen levels. Also, drugs containing azo dyes will have a masking effect on the urobilinogen area.

QUALITATIVE EHRLICH'S TEST

Prior to the introduction of the semiquantitative UROBILISTIX® reagent strip test, Ehrlich's test was the routine procedure for determining urobilinogen.

1. Place 10 ml urine in a test tube. Allow to warm to room temperature.
2. Add 1 ml Ehrlich's reagent and mix.
3. Let stand 3 to 5 minutes.
4. Normal amounts of urobilinogen present in the urine sample will change the solution to pink color, observable when viewed from

top of the test tube against a white background placed beneath the bottom of the test tube. Abnormally high amounts of urobilinogen will change the solution to a clearly discernible cherry red color.

Ehrlich's reagent is prepared as follows:

Paradimethylaminobenzaldehyde	10 gm
hydrochloric acid, concentrated	75 ml
water	75 ml

QUALITATIVE SCHLESSINGER TEST
1. Place 10 ml urine in a test tube.
2. Add 10 ml of a saturated alcoholic solution of zinc acetate (10 gm zinc acetate suspended in 100 ml ethanol).
3. Mix and filter.
4. Separate filtrate equally into 2 test tubes.
5. Add 1 drop concentrated HCl to one tube only.
6. Add 2 drops Lugol's solution (5 gm iodine, 10 gm potassium iodide dissolved in 100 ml water) to each tube. Mix by inversion.
7. View tubes for fluorescence with a Wood's light. Urobilinogen will produce a green-yellow fluorescence in the unacidified tube alone. Porphyrins produce red fluorescence.

Quantitative urobilinogen determinations are complex chemical procedures requiring the use of a colorimeter or spectrophotometer. For most routine chemical and diagnostic purposes, the semiquantitative test with the reagent strips described above is adequate.

2 hour Test for Urobilinogen—Watson
1. Record the total 2 hour volume of urine.
2. Place 3 ml urine in a colorimeter tube.
3. Add 3 ml Ehrlich's reagent strip and mix.
   This reagent is prepared as follows:

paradimethylaminobenzaldehyde	0.7 gm
hydrochloric acid, concentrated	150 ml
distilled water	100 ml

4. Add 6 ml saturated solution of sodium acetate and mix.
5. Read immediately in a spectrophotometer because the color development is unstable. The spectrophotometer is standardized with a blank solution containing a colorless mixture in which 3 ml Ehrlich's reagent were added to 6 ml saturated sodium acetate, mixed, and then 3 ml urine added and mixed again.
6. The amount of urobilinogen is calculated from a calibration curve made from standardized solutions of known quantities of urobilinogen or Pontacyl dyes. The answer is recorded in terms of Ehrlich units rather than quantity of urobilinogen because Ehrlich's solution reacts with chromogens other than urobilinogen in the urine. These substances, however, increase proportionally with urobilinogen.

DETECTION OF BACTERIURIA

15.

The finding of bacteria in a random urine can be considered indicative of a urinary tract infection only if the specimen is a clean-voided midstream sample collected under aseptic conditions in a sterile container that is immediately closed with a sterile cap. Meticulous care must be exercised during collection and afterward to avoid contamination of the urine specimen with incidental organisms or potential pathogens from sources external to the urinary tract. Preferably, testing for bacteriuria should begin within an hour from the time of urine collection, but if this is not possible, the specimen should be refrigerated at 5° C immediately after collection and tested within eight hours. Under no circumstances should a preservative be added to urine intended for bacteriological culture tests. The preferable type of specimen is first morning urine or if this is not practical, urine that has incubated in the bladder at least four hours. See Chapter 3 for detailed description of proper methods for obtaining a urine sample to be tested for bacteriuria.

CLINICAL UTILITY

The concentration of bacteria in urine generally serves to distinguish between urinary tract infection and contamination of the specimen. As a result of correlating numerous laboratory findings with clinical conditions, a "critical level" of bacterial concentration is now generally used in evaluating the clinical significance of bacteriuria.

Bacteriuria is considered *significant* when laboratory findings show the presence of 100,000 (10^5) or more bacteria per ml. of the urine specimen. If contamination of an otherwise "sterile specimen" with bacteria from external sources has occurred, the count may be as low as 10,000 (10^4) or even 1,000 (10^3) or less per ml. When the count is between 10^3 and 10^5, the possibility of an incipient urinary tract infection is suggested, and in such cases the physician may request that another clean-voided midstream urine specimen be obtained for repeat testing.

Even a very low count of bacteria is sufficient to confirm the diagnosis when clinical symptoms of urinary tract infection are also present. Low counts may occur in patients with frank urinary tract infections if the urine specimen is very dilute or has remained in the bladder only a short time. Such counts may also occur during early stages of treatment with an antimicrobial agent.

Significant urinary tract infections may be present in patients who have experienced no symptoms. Despite absence of symptoms, these infections are serious because they have the potential for causing severe kidney damage before the patient is aware of them. This condition is known as a *significant asymptomatic bacteriuria* and can be defined as the finding of 10^5 or more bacteria per ml. of urine in the absence of clinical symptoms. With the recent advent of simpler, less expensive methods for detecting and semiquantitating bacteriuria, more and more physicians are finding it worthwhile to request bacteriuria tests for high-risk types of patients even though symptoms are absent. High-risk types include pregnant patients, school children (especially girls), diabetic patients, and patients with a previous history of urinary tract infections.

Gram-negative bacteria of the types normally present in the large intestine are the organisms most commonly identified in urinary tract infections. Of these, *Escherichia coli, Proteus species, Klebsiella,* and *Pseudomonas aeruginosa* are found most frequently. Gram-positive organisms such as *Streptococcus faecalis* and *Staphylococcus aureus* cause infections somewhat less frequently.

DETERMINATIONS

Several methods are available for detecting and semiquantitating bacteria in the urine. They range from microscopic examination and chemical tests to recently developed culture strip techniques that are especially suited to use in the urinalysis laboratory. Conventional agar-plate culture techniques for precise quantitation and identification of bacterial species and strains are outside the scope of this book since they require training and experience in microbiology and the facilities of a microbiology laboratory.

MICROSCOPIC EXAMINATION

The *centrifuged sediment,* when examined microscopically as part of the general urinalysis, can reveal bacteria if present. Most of the important "rods" are especially easy to identify, the coccal forms are a little more difficult. The finding of 20 or more bacteria per high power field may indicate a urinary tract infection, while the presence of only a few bacteria should be interpreted with caution, possibly suggesting a urinary tract infection that cannot be confirmed or excluded until more definitive studies are performed.

SIMPLIFIED, SEMIQUANTITATIVE CULTURE TESTS

The urinalysis laboratory can now use convenient, easy-to-interpret culture tests for detecting and semiquantitating bacteriuria with greater precision than possible with nitrite tests. Several types of reagent strips or glass slides coated with agar are available; they are dipped in urine, inserted in a sterile container, and incubated at 37° C. Colonies are counted or appearance is compared with a reference chart 12 to 24 hours later. Many of these have the disadvantage of requiring continuous storage before use in a refrigerator, and some are sufficiently bulky to require a standard incubator if numerous tests are being done simultaneously.

MICROSTIX®-3 Reagent Strips, a *3-way bacteriuria test* contains a nitrite reagent pad and two dehydrated culture media pads. One of the latter favors growth of all bacterial types commonly found in urinary tract infections while the other supports growth of only Gram-negative types.

In using this 3-way test, the MICROSTIX®-3 strip is removed from its wrapper, taking care not to touch or otherwise contaminate the test areas. The strip is dipped in the urine specimen for five seconds and removed. The nitrite test is read 30 seconds later, any degree of pink color suggesting the presence of 10^5 or more organisms per ml of urine. The strip is then inserted and sealed in the sterile plastic pouch provided, incubated for 12 to 18 hours, and the results read without removing from the transparent pouch. Magenta-colored spots on the culture media pads represent bacterial locations, and the density of these spots is compared with the chart provided. If bacteria are present, this comparison shows the degree of concentration (10^1, 10^2, 10^3, 10^4 or 10^5 or more bacteria per ml) of Gram-negative and total bacteria.

Since the culture media pads on MICROSTIX®-3 are dehydrated, refrigeration is not required, and the product is stable at room temperature. A small, inexpensive, thermostatically controlled incubator designed specifically for incubation of MICROSTIX®-3 makes this bacteriuria testing system highly practical for the urinalysis laboratory. The incubator occupies about the same space on a table or laboratory bench as an average textbook, and yet it accommodates 30 pouches. By reading the results of the culture test without removing the MICROSTIX®-3 strip from the sealed transparent pouch, dispersal of potentially dangerous pathogens into the laboratory environment is avoided. After results are read and recorded, the still-sealed pouches are easily and safely disposed of by incineration.

A *stained smear of uncentrifuged or centrifuged urine* can also be examined under the oil immersion lens to detect bacteriuria. The finding of bacteria on the smear suggests significant bacteriuria. The technique consists of allowing a drop of urine to air-dry on a microscopic slide. After it is heat-fixed in a flame, it is stained with Gram's stain or methlene blue stain (Wright's stain). Gram's stain, although slightly more complex in its method of use, is considered superior for identification of bacteria.

Technique for Gram's Stain
1. Cover slide for 1 minute with 1% crystal violet.
2. Wash with water.
3. Cover with Gram's iodine solution for 30 seconds
   iodine   1.0 gm
   potassium iodide   2.0 gm
   distilled water   300 ml
4. Decolorize with 95% ethyl alcohol or acetone until no more dye runs off slide.
5. Counterstain with dilute safranin for 30 seconds. Wash and dry.

CHEMICAL TESTS

Several types of chemical tests have been used to detect bacteriuria, including determination of glucose consumption, activity of specific enymes, reduction of triphenyltetrazolium chloride, and reduction of uriary nitrates to nitrites. With the exception of the nitrite test, chemical screening has not proved practical for general use.

The nitrite test is both inexpensive and rapid, and it provides an ndirect method for early detection of significant bacteriuria. Common nfecting organisms such as species of Enterobacter, Citrobacter, Escheichia, Proteus, Klebsiella, and Pseudomonas contain enzymes that reduce nitrate in the urine to nitrite. Urinalysis test strips like N-MULTISTIX®, N-URISTIX®, MICROSTIX®-Nitrite, and MICROSTIX®-3 Reagent Strip contain reagent areas that change color in the presence of nitrite.

Any degree of uniform pink color should be interpreted as a positive nitrite test suggesting the presence of 10^5 or more organisms per ml, but color development is not proportional to the number of bacteria present.

Thus a positive result from a nitrite screening test would seem to be an indication of significant bacteriuria. However, *a negative test result should never be interpreted as indicating absence of bacteriuria;* there are several reasons for this.

First morning urine or urine that has remained in the bladder for several hours is more likely to yield a positive nitrite test result in the presence of significant bacteriuria than a random urine sample that may have been in the bladder only a short time. In the latter type of specimen, there may have been insufficient time for the conversion of nitrate to nitrite to have occurred. There are rare instances in which nitrate does not appear in the urine, and a patient of this type could have significant bacteriuria without a positive nitrite test. Some strains of urinary pathogens do not produce the enzymes necessary to reduce nitrate to nitrite— another reason there may be significant bacteriuria despite a negative nitrite test. (Table 5)

Table 5

ORGANISMS THAT DO REDUCE NITRATE TO NITRITE
1. E. coli
2. Klebsiella pneumoniae
3. Enterobacter aerogenes
4. Proteus species
5. Pseudomonas species (some strains)
6. Edwardsiella species
7. Serratia marcescens
8. Salmonella (some strains)
9. Shigella species
10. Citrobacter species
11. Most Staphylococcus

ORGANISMS THAT DO NOT REDUCE NITRATES TO NITRITES
1. Streptococcus faecalis
2. Gonococcus
3. Tuberculosis

INSTRUMENTATION IN URINE CHEMISTRY

16.

Recent developments in technology has led to instrumentation in automation and semi-automation of urine chemistry tests. Automated and semi-automated urinalysis techniques have been needed in the laboratory for sometime. Some reasons for instrumentation are:

1. Large numbers of urine specimens.
2. Lack of standardization in strip reading.
3. Lack of precision of reproducibility from reader to reader.

CLINILAB®

The CLINILAB® (Figure 15) automates urine chemistry by automatically mixing, dispensing, performing pH, protein, glucose, ketone, blood, bilirubin, urobilinogen, specific gravity, and then printing the final results on a patient identification card, or the results may be interfaced directly into a computer. Specific gravity is performed by the so called "falling

CLINILAB®

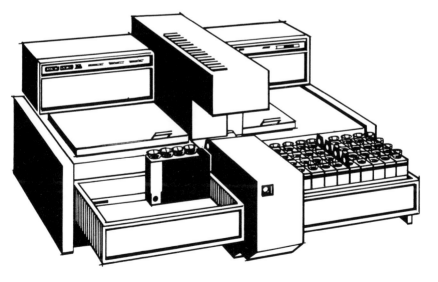

Figure 15

65

drop" method discussed in Chapter 5. The CLINILAB® is designed to test two urines per minute and is useful in laboratories performing over 200 specimens per day.

The results obtained from CLINILAB® are from the same solid-state reagent areas used on the AMES multiple reagent strips. Also, most human errors of misrecording and misidentification are minimized by using CLINILAB®.

CLINI-TEK®

CLINI-TEK® (Figure 16) is a semi-automated reflectance photometer to read AMES multiple urinalysis reagent strips. CLINI-TEK® "reads," displays or prints results of urine pH, protein, glucose, ketone, bilirubin, blood, nitrite, urobilinogen and specific gravity.

By using a unique optics system and microprocessor technology, the instrument measures the light energy reflected from the reacting reagent area. The CLINI-TEK® is calibrated with a dry urine strip and a positive reference solution at least once daily. The operator then dips a reagent strip into a mixed specimen, withdraws it and simultaneously activates the CLINI-TEK®. The strip is then placed on the feed table with the reagent areas facing up, drawn into the CLINI-TEK® and read. As reflectance is read, the appropriate value is displayed or printed for each reagent area on the strip.

CLINI-TEK®

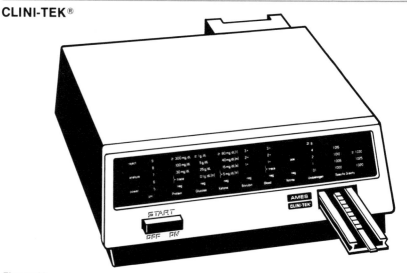

Figure 16.

Automated and semi-automated urine chemistry allows for elimination of the variable that has commonly caused erroneous and confusing results when color has been interpreted by the human eye.

PHENYLPRUVIC ACID (PKU) AND PORPHYRINS IN URINE

17.

PHENYLPYRUVIC ACID

A disease known as *phenylketonuria,* or *PKU,* is first manifested by the presence of phenylpyruvic acid in the urine. It is caused by hereditary absence of the enzyme, phenylalanine hydroxylase, essential for converting phenylalanine to tyrosine in its normal pathway of metabolism. Thus, the phenylalanine ingested in milk and other foods accumulates in the tissues and blood. By the age of four weeks and often much earlier, intermediate metabolites of phenylalanine, particularly phenylpyruvic acid, begin appearing in the infant's urine. When untreated, PKU results in brain damage and severe mental retardation. However, when detected early and treated with a diet low in phenylalanine, the prognosis is good for normal mental development. Therefore, testing the blood or urine of infants frequently during early life is one of the most convenient ways of detecting phenylketonuria.

METHODS OF DETERMINATION

PHENISTIX® Reagent Strips are impregnated with a solution containing ferric ions that form a specific bluish gray to gray-green color reaction with phenylpyruvic acid. The strips are buffered to prevent interference from phosphates. The strip is either dipped into a fresh sample of urine or pressed against a wet diaper. After exactly 30 seconds, it is compared to a color chart scaled at concentrations of 0, 15 mg, 40 mg, and 100 mg phenylpyruvic acid per 100 ml urine.

PHENISTIX® turn a pink to purple color in urine containing salicylates and phenothiazine derivatives. Also high concentrations of bilirubin or ammonia in the urine alter the normal color reaction developed with phenylpyruvic acid.

The *ferric chloride test* forms color reactions that can be used to detect phenylketonuria.

To perform the rest:

1. Add 2 drops of dilute hydrochloric acid to 5 ml of urine to acidify the urine.
2. Add 2 drops of 10% ferric chloride solution and observe for color formation. A dark green, transient color that fades to yellow signifies phenylpyruvic acid. A red to purple color occurs with salicylates, acetylphenetidines, phenol, and phenothiazide derivatives.

Phosphate ions in the urine may cause a false negative result. They can be removed before performing the test by first taking:

1. 1 ml of magnesium reagent (11 gm $MgCl_2$, 14 gm NH_4Cl, 20.0 ml conc. NH_4OH; dilute to 1 liter with water).
2. Add to 4.0 ml urine and mix.
3. Let stand 5 minutes; filter.
4. Then perform the ferric chloride test.

PORPHYRINS

Porphyrins are cyclic tetrapyrrole compounds, some of which are found in erythrocytes, some of which are precursors of heme, and some of which the body uses to synthesize the respiratory enzymes, the cytochromes. These compounds are pigments or precursors of pigments and their presence turns urine a pink to red color. The urine of patients with porphyria usually is deep red in color but may vary from pale pink to almost black. Some patients excrete urine of normal color which subsequently turns dark after exposure to light.

REFERENCE VALUES

Coproporphyrins are normally excreted in the urine in amounts ranging from 70 to 250 μg/day. Uroporphyrin excretion in the urine normally ranges from 10 to 30 μg/day, porphobilinogen excretion does not exceed 2 mg/day, and delta-aminolevulinic acid excretion is between 1.0 and 7.0 mg/day.

CLINICAL UTILITY

INBORN ERRORS OF METABOLISM

In diseases involving hepatic metabolism, excessive production of porphyrins occurs in the liver.

In *acute intermittent porphyria,* the liver produces an excessive amount of porphyrin precursors, primarily porphobilinogen and delta-aminolevulinic acid. Clinical symptoms include intermittent severe ab-

dominal pain and neurologic manifestations such as peripheral neuro-
pathy, bulbar symptoms, psychotic alterations in personality, and
involvement of the autonomic nervous system. The onset of the disease
is usually after puberty. The urine may darken on standing due to conversion of porphobilinogen to porphobilin and uroporphyrin. Acute exacerbations may be precipitated by alcohol, barbiturates, and hepatotoxins.

Porphyria cutanea tarda is caused by defects in porphyrin metabo-
ism in the liver. It is characterized by attacks of acute abdominal colic
and by skin manifestations beginning between ages 10 and 30. The skin
develops bullous lesions when exposed to sunlight or after mechanical
trauma. Excretion of porphobilinogen and delta-aminolevulinic acid in
the urine is increased during times of acute exacerbations; it is normal at
other times. Coproporphyrin and uroporphyrin excretion in the urine is
increased during acute attacks; coproporphyrin and protoporphyrin excretion in the feces is increased at all times. During acute attacks, the
urine is red in color.

In diseases involving erythrocyte metabolism, excessive amounts of
porphyrins are synthesized in erythrocytes in the bone marrow.

Congenital erythropoietic porphyria is a disease that becomes man-
ifest in infancy with the onset of sensitivity to sunlight, formation of large
bullous lesions over the exposed skin areas, and increased hemolysis
and erythropoiesis. The urine is pink to red in color and contains increased amounts of uroporphyrin I and coproporphyrin I.

ACQUIRED DISORDERS OF PORPHYRIN METABOLISM

Acquired porphyria cutanea tarda occurs in patients with disorders
of liver metabolism such as alcoholic and nutritional liver cirrhosis, exposure to certain hepatotoxic chemical agents, and liver malignancies.
Clinical manifestations are the same as found in congenital porphyria
cutanea tarda, and increased urinary excretion of uroporphyrin and coproporphyrin occurs.

Elevated coproporphyrin excretion in the urine occurs in many diseases: infections, malignancies, alcoholic cirrhosis, infectious hepatitis,
and obstructive jaundice.

In *lead poisoning,* coproporphyrin III excretion in the urine is markedly elevated beyond the range that occurs in any other type of disease.
Coproporphyrin excretion may rise from a norm of up to 250 μg/day to 40
times as high, about 10 mg/day. Measurement of coproporphyrin III levels
is especially important for the diagnosis and daily clinical management
of patients with lead poisoning.

DETERMINATIONS

Screening tests are available for the indentification of porphobilinogen and coproporphyrin.

Porphobilinogen—Watson-Schwartz Test
1. Place 2.5 ml fresh urine in a test tube.
2. Add 2.5 ml Ehrlich's reagent and mix.

paradimethylaminobenzaldehyde	3.5 gm
hydrochloric acid, concentrated	750 ml
distilled water	500 ml

3. Add 5 ml saturated sodium acetate (1 kg sodium acetate dissolved in 1 L water at 60° C.) and mix well.
4. A pink-red color appearing at this time indicates porphobilinogen or other Ehrlich reacting substances such as urobilinogen.
5. Add 5 ml chloroform, shake, and either centrifuge or allow to stand and settle out.
6. The chloroform layer goes to the bottom, carrying with it urobilinogen and other Ehrlich reacting substances.
7. If porphobilinogen is present, the upper layer will turn a deep red or red-purple color.

Coproporphyrin Test to Detect Lead Poisoning
1. Place 5 ml urine in test tube.
2. Add 1.0 ml glacial acetic acid.
3. Then add 5 ml ethyl ether.
4. Add 3 drops of fresh 3% hydrogen peroxide.
5. Stopper test tube. Mix by inversion 8 to 12 times.
6. Let stand for 10 to 15 minutes until either layer separates.
7. Examine tube in a darkened room with ultraviolet reflected light (Wood's light) to detect fluorescence in the topmost, ether layer. Pale blue fluorescence signifies negative or normal amounts of coproporphyrins in urine. Fluorescence ranging in color from violet and pink to light rose and then dark rose indicates, successively, a 1+ through 4+ concentration of coproporphyrin.

MICROSCOPIC EXAMINATION OF URINE SEDIMENT

18.

A qualitative or semiquantitative evaluation of urine sediment generally provides adequate information for the majority of diagnostic and clinical needs. Quantitative examination of the urine is most helpful in evaluating the course and progression of renal disease.

Microscopic examination of urine sediment can provide the following information:

1. Evidence of renal disease as opposed to lower urinary tract infection.
2. Indicate the type and state of activity of a renal lesion or disease condition.

The microscopic result and urine chemistry result should be checked against each other before reports are issued.

Urine sediment examination is considered the most inaccurate and imprecise procedure in routine urinalysis because of the many variations in preparation technique. Standardization of variables, such as urine volume, centrifugation time and speed, and volume of urine sediment examined, is necessary to achieve reliable and reproducible results.

QUALITATIVE TECHNIQUE

Examination of the sediment is more reliable when the urine is concentrated. If the specimen is too dilute, the cellular elements may be lysed and the amount of sediment obtained for examination, even after centrifugation, may not be representative. The urine must be freshly voided and examined without excessive delay in order to prevent cellular deterioration. Cellular debris from the urethral meatus and secretions from the vagina may contaminate the urine specimen.

To obtain the sediment, 10 to 15 ml of urine should be taken from a freshly mixed urine specimen and centrifuged at a standard speed, usually 1500 to 2000 rpm for 5 minutes. The supernatant fluid is poured off and the sediment resuspended in 1 ml of the same fluid. If the sediment is sparse, it should be examined with little or no additional dilution.

A drop of the resuspended sediment is placed directly on a microscope slide and covered with a coverslip. The slide is first examined under low power magnification to locate casts and elements that are present in only a few fields. Casts tend to congregate near the edges of the coverslip. After the entire slide has been scanned, a further examination is made under high power (dry) magnification in order to identify specific types of cells, crystals, elements, and objects present in the urine and to delineate the various types of casts. A minimum of 10 to 15 high power fields should be scanned for this examination. Good technique requires varying the intensity of the light source of the microscope in order to correctly identify the various components of the sediment. Some elements are more easily recognized in subdued light, others in brighter light.

Red blood cells, leucocytes, and epithelial cells are conventionally reported in terms of cells per high power field; casts are counted per low power field. For each determination, the number of elements seen in at least 10 fields should be counted and the average of this number used for the reported value. Other elements, such as bacteria, parasites, crystals, and spermatozoa, are usually reported as well. This method for preparing the sediment and counting the elements converts the microscopic analysis of random urine specimens from a qualitative description of the sediment to a semiquantitative estimation of the numbers of cells and casts present in the specimens and their relative frequencies.

STAINS

The sediment usually is examined unstained as this technique generally provides adequate information for routine use. If a stain is desired several are available. A procedure for the STERNHEIMER stain for urine sediment is given below.

STERNHEIMER STAIN[8]

FORMULA FOR STAIN

National fast blue (Allied Chemical Corp., No. 1946P), list 2% aqueous solution, filtered.
Pyronin B (Matheson Coleman & Bell No. Pb17), 1.5% solution, filtered

Note: It may be necessary to purify the pyronin by alcohol extraction to standardize dye content. Mix equal parts of National fast blue and Pyronin B.

STAINING THE SEDIMENT
1. Add 2 drops of stain mixture to 1 drop of urine sediment. Mix thoroughly by flicking tube with finger.
2. Place 1 drop of stained sediment on clean slide. Cover slip.

STAIN CHARACTERISTICS

Leukocytes may appear unstained initially, or the nucleus may appear red-blue with red cytoplasm after a prolonged period of time. Hyaline casts stain bright blue, while finely granular casts stain bright red. Coarsely granular casts stain reddish violet, "waxy casts" also stain reddish violet. RBC casts are outlined in shades of pink while hemoglobin casts appear rust brown. Miscellaneous substances such as oval fat bodies and yeast will not stain. Trichomonas, if present, will not stain, or may appear bluish.

NORMAL SEDIMENT

Normal sediment is not free of cells or casts but contains a limited number of formed elements. A precise definition of normalcy is difficult to obtain, but the presence of one or two blood cells per high power field, one or two leucocytes and a few epithelial cells is not necessarily considered abnormal. The urine of mature females may also contain large numbers of squamous epithelial cells from the vaginal walls. An occasional hyaline cast may also be a normal finding.

SEDIMENT IN DISEASE—CLINICAL SIGNIFICANCE

RED BLOOD CELLS

The finding of more than one or two red blood cells per high power field is an abnormal condition. It can indicate a variety of renal and systemic diseases, including trauma to the kidney. It may also be found following violent exercise. It may follow traumatic catheterization, the passage of stones, or contamination from menstrual blood. Hematuria occurs with pyelonephritis, tuberculosis of the genitourinary tract, cystitis, prostatitis, renal calculi, renal tumors, and other malignancies of the urinary tract, and hemorrhagic diseases such as hemophilia, etc. Red blood cells will tend to lyse or dissolve if allowed to stand in urine which is alkaline or dilute.

WHITE BLOOD CELLS

The presence of large numbers of white cells (leucocytes) usually indicates bacterial infection in the urinary tract. Pyuria may also be seen in acute glomerulonephritis. The cells are segmented neutrophils or "polys". Large amounts of mononuclear cells "Lymphs", in a patient with a kidney transplant may indicate early tissue rejection phenomena.

EPITHELIAL CELLS

Large numbers of renal epithelial cells may indicate active tubular degeneration. These cells are noted in the urine of patients with acute tubular necrosis and necrotizing papillitis. Squamous epithelial cells appear frequently in normal urine. Figure 17 shows the origin of various epithelial cells which may appear in the urine. However, due to the osmotic, pH and traumatic changes the cells undergo during passage through the genitourinary system, they rarely retain their original shape.

EPITHELIAL CELLS IN URINE

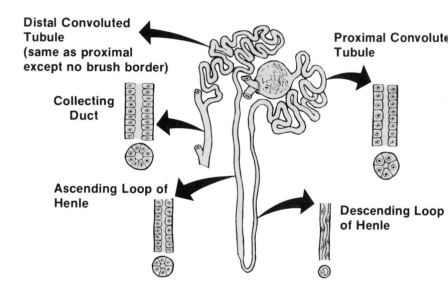

Distal Convoluted Tubule (same as proximal except no brush border)

Proximal Convolute Tubule

Collecting Duct

Ascending Loop of Henle

Descending Loop of Henle

Figure 17

CRYSTALS

The type and quantity of crystalline precipitate vary with the pH of the urine. Amorphous material is of little importance. Crystals in normal urine are formed as the specimen cools. Crystals of abnormal urine include cystine, leucine and tyrosine, and cholesterin. Table 6 lists some crystals found in urine sediment and the physical-chemical characteristics associated with them.

Table 6

INORGANIC SEDIMENT: **ACID URINE**

NAME	COLOR	SHAPE	ALK	ACID	ALCOHOL	°C	OTHER
				SOLUBILITY			
Amorphous urates	Brick-Red	Granules	+	−	−	60°C	Acetic Acid
Uric Acid	Yellow-Brown	Polymorphous—whetstones, rosettes of prisms, rhombohedral prisms, hexagonal plate	+	−	−	−	−
Sodium urate	Colorless to Yellow	Fan of slender prisms	+	−	−	60°C	−
Cystine (rare)	1) Colorless 2) Highly refractile	Flat hexagonal plates with well-defined edges Singly or in clusters	+	+	−	−	−
Cholesterol (rare)	1) Colorless	"Broken window panes" with notched corners Flat plates	−	−	+	−	Ether Chloroform
Leucine (rare)	1) Yellow or Brown 2) Highly refractile	Spheroids with striations Pure form hexagonal	+	−	+	−	Slightly in hot H_2O
Tyrosine (rare)	Colorless or Yellow	Fine silky needles in sheaves or rosettes	+	+	−	−	−
Bilirubin	Reddish Brown	Cubes Rhombic plates Amorphous needles	+	+	−	60°C	Acetone Chloroform
ACID, NEUTRAL, OR SLIGHTLY ALKALINE URINE							
Calcium oxalate	Colorless	Octahedral Dumbells Often small—use h.p.	−	+	−	−	Dilute HCl
Hippuric acid	Colorless	Rhombic plates Four sided prisms	+	−	−	−	Hot H_2O
ALKALINE, NEUTRAL, OR SLIGHTLY ACID URINE							
Triple phosphate	Colorless	"Coffin lids" 3-6 sided prism Occ. fern-leaf	−	−	−	−	Dilute Acetic Acid
ALKALINE URINE							
Calcium carbonate	Colorless	Needles Spheres Dumbells	−	−	−	−	Acetic Acid
Ammonium biurate	Yellow Opaque Brown	"Thorn apple" spheres Dumbells Sheaves of needles	+	−	−	60°C with Acetic Acid	−
Calcium phosphate	Colorless	Prisms Plates Needles	−	−	−	−	Dilute Acetic Acid

75

BACTERIA

Normal urine contains no bacteria. If proper and careful technique was used to obtain the sample and if the specimen was protected from contaminants before the examination, the presence of bacteria in significant numbers may indicate urinary tract infection. The presence of leucocytes helps to differentiate between "contamination" and a "true infection."

YEAST AND PARASITES

Yeast cells (Candida albicans) may be indicative of urinary moniliasis, especially in patients with diabetes mellitus. Frequently, yeast appears as a contaminant in the urine of female patients with vaginal moniliasis.

The majority of parasites observed in urine are contaminants from fecal or vaginal material. A urinary tract parasite infestation may be associated with the presence of red blood cells, as in *Schistosoma haematobium.*

SPERMATOZOA

Spermatozoa are frequently seen in the urine following nocturnal emissions or sexual intercourse.

CASTS

Cast formation occurs usually in the distal convoluted tubule of the nephron. Casts may also occur in the ascending loop of Henle or the collecting duct. Requirements for cast formation are an acid condition, high salt concentration, reduced urine flow, and protein. (Figure 18)

Casts are named according to the matrix of the inclusions contained in them, e.g. red blood cell cast, white blood cell cast, etc.

Red blood cell casts indicate the presence of an acute inflammatory or vascular disorder in the glomerulus causing renal hematuria. They should always be regarded as pathological and may be the only manifestation of acute glomerulonephritis, renal infarction, collagen disease, or kidney involvement in subacute bacterial endocarditis. *White blood cell casts* may be found in the urine from patients with acute glomerulonephritis, nephrotic syndrome, or pyelonephritis.

Since pyelonephritis may remain completely asymptomatic even though it is progressively destroying renal tissue, careful examination of the urinary sediment for leucocyte casts is important. In some cases it may be the only significant laboratory finding in an asymptomatic situation. *Epithelial cell casts* are formed by fused desquamated tubular cells. Since the tubule is a living membrane, it is always replacing itself. Thus, the finding of an occasional renal epithelial cell or clump is not remarkable. However, in any disease producing damage to tubular epithelium, the appearance of many epithelial casts may indicate excessive desquamation such as may occur in nephrosis, eclampsia, amyloidosis, and in the

CAST FORMATION

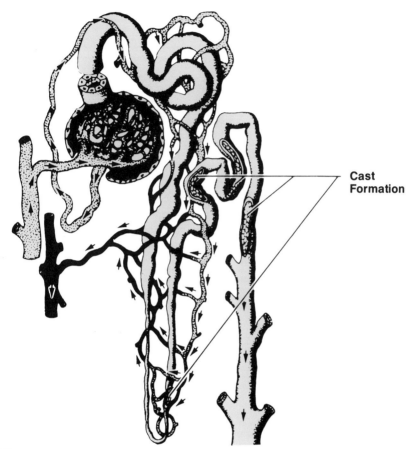

Cast
Formation

Figure 18

presence of poisoning with heavy metals and a variety of other toxins. *Hyaline casts,* formed of the gel of Tamm-Horsfall protein, imply damage to the glomerular capillary membrane, permitting leakage of proteins through the glomerular filter. Such damage may be permanent or transient as a result of fever or the effects of posture (orthostatic, lordotic), emotional stress, or strenuous exercise.

Granular casts—The terms "coarsely granular" and "finely granular" are merely descriptive, indicating the degree of degeneration that has occurred in the cellular inclusion—the cells having been broken down into coarse or finer particles. While an occasional granular cast may be found in normal individuals, their presence beyond an "occasional cast" may indicate pyelonephritis. Granular casts are also found in chronic lead intoxication.

Waxy and fatty casts—These casts are associated with tubular inflammation and degeneration. The broad, waxy cast is formed in the collecting tubules when the urine flow through them is reduced. Both waxy and fatty casts are found in chronic renal disease.

IDENTIFICATION OF SPECIFIC ELEMENTS IN THE SEDIMENT

RED BLOOD CELLS

Red blood cells usually look like pale, light refractive, biconcave discs when viewed under high power magnification. They have no nuclei. Red blood cells seen in fresh, unstained sediment are pale in color; in urine that is not fresh, they are pale or colorless "shadow cells"; in concentrated urine, they may be small and crenated; and in dilute urine, they are often large and swollen and sometimes rupture to produce "ghost" cells. Red blood cells must be differentiated from yeast cells, urate crystals, and oil droplets. Yeast cells are usually ovoid and frequently show budding. Ammonium biurate crystals occur in large quantities with great range in the size of crystals. Mineral oil droplets also vary greatly in their size and are more refractile and spherical. (Figure 19)

ERYTHROCYTES, High power

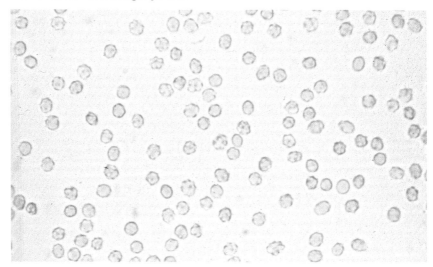

Figure 19

WHITE CELLS

The predominant type of leucocyte (Fig. 20) appearing in the urine is the polymorphonuclear leucocyte. It is sometimes difficult to differentiate this cell from the various types of epithelial cells because of deterioration of cell structure prior to the examination. Therefore, these cells usually are estimated as one entity in both the qualitative and quantitative analysis of the urinary sediment. The leucocytes have segmented nuclei, are usually granular, and are approximately 1½ times as large as red blood cells. Certain neutrophils are larger than the usual leucocytes, and their cytoplasmic granules have Brownian movements. These cells are called granular motility or "glitter" cells. Originally they were thought to be pathognomic of pyelonephritis, but are now thought to be a result of hypotonic urine.

LEUCOCYTES, High power

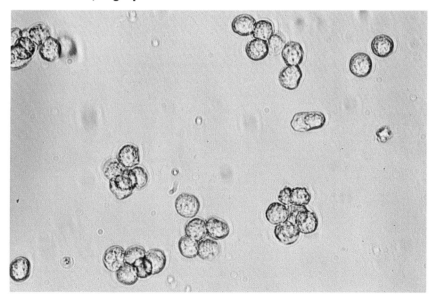

Figure 20

EPITHELIAL CELLS

Renal tubular epithelial cells are round and are slightly larger than leucocytes. Each contains a single large nucleus.

Bladder epithelial cells are larger than renal tubular epithelial cells. They range in shape from flat, to cuboidal, and then columnar.

79

Squamous epithelial cells are large flat cells with single small nuclei and a large cytoplasm. The majority of these cells are contaminants from the vagina or vulva, but some originate in the urethra. (Figure 21)

SQUAMOUS EPITHELIAL CELLS AND ERYTHROCYTES

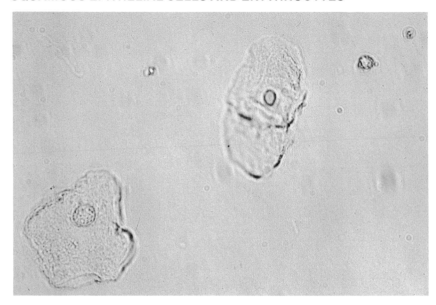

Figure 21

CASTS

The appearance of a cast, its size and its inclusion will offer incontrovertible evidence of the condition of at least one nephron of one kidney just prior to passage of the urine.

Practically all casts have a hyaline matrix, which may or may not contain inclusions such as desquamated cells from the lining of tubules, pus cells or red blood cells. Casts are classified according to the contained material.

Red blood cell casts form in three stages: (1) presence of free red cells; (2) degenerating cells within a protein matrix; (3) homogeneous blood casts. (Figure 22)

- Any Disease which Alters the Integrity of the Glomerulus will alter the Composition of the Urine
- Disease or Injury to the Glomerulus usually results in a Leakage of RBCs and Protein

80

FORMATION OF RED BLOOD CELL CAST

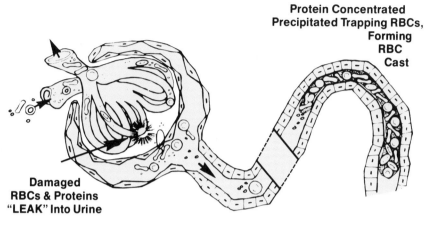

Protein Concentrated Precipitated Trapping RBCs, Forming RBC Cast

Damaged RBCs & Proteins "LEAK" Into Urine

Figure 22

An actual photograph of a red blood cell cast is shown in Figure 23.

RED BLOOD CELL CAST

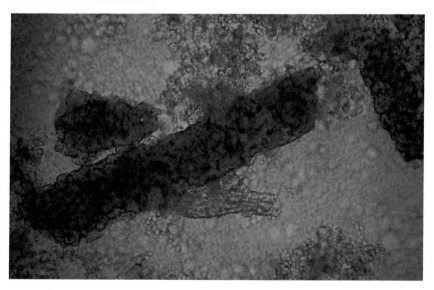

Figure 23

White cell casts are usually composed of many leucocytes in a cylindrical encasement and indicate renal origin. Figure 24 shows the formation of a white blood cell cast.

- Interstitial Diseases—Pyelonephritis, An Intrarenal Infection caused by a Gram-Negative Microorganism (usually), which may enter from the blood stream (septicemia) or from infections in the bladder and/or urethra

FORMATION OF WHITE BLOOD CELL CAST

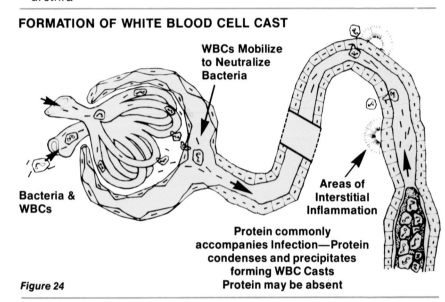

WBCs Mobilize
to Neutralize
Bacteria

Bacteria &
WBCs

Areas of
Interstitial
Inflammation

Protein commonly
accompanies Infection—Protein
condenses and precipitates
forming WBC Casts
Protein may be absent

Figure 24

A typical white blood cell cast seen in the urine sediment is shown in Figure 25.

WHITE BLOOD CELL CAST, Low power

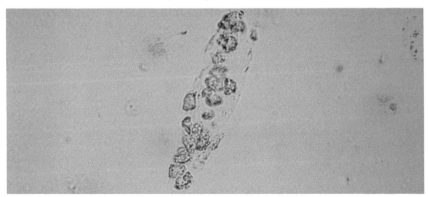

Figure 25

Coarse granular casts contain homogeneous coarsely granular material. They are clear, colorless and dense appearing. Coarse granular casts may represent the initial stages of degeneration of epithelial cell casts. These casts further degenerate into fine granular casts and terminate as waxy casts, or fatty casts, if replacement with fat occurred initially.

Fine granular casts are differentiated from coarse granular casts by the presence of fine granular material. Figure 26 shows several typical granular casts.

GRANULAR CAST, Low power

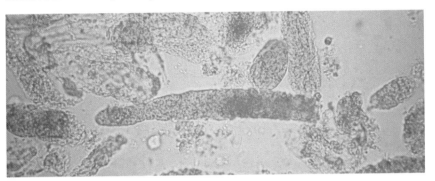

Figure 26

Waxy casts are composed of a homogeneous, yellowish material. They are relatively broad, have a highly refractile outline, and appear very brittle. They are irregularly shaped, show characteristic clefts and occasionally may have a "corkscrew" appearance. (Figure 27)

WAXY CASTS, High power

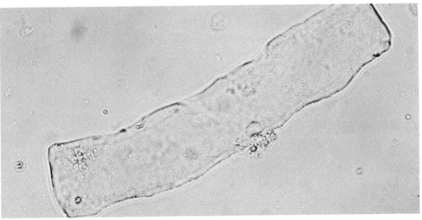

Figure 27

Broad casts (renal failure casts) are from two to six times as wide as ordinary casts. They are usually waxy, granular, or cellular. They are thought to arise in the collecting tubules as a result of markedly decreased urinary output, presumably due to severe renal disease. (Figure 28)

BROAD CAST, High power (waxy)

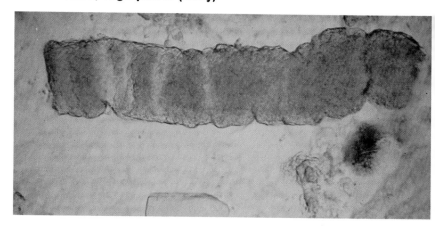

Figure 28

Epithelial cell casts are formed by fused desquamated tubular cells. The degeneration of the discrete cellular casts into coarsely and finely granular material is purely a function of age and permits the inference that there has been stasis in the nephron. (Figure 29)

EPITHELIAL CELL CAST, 200X

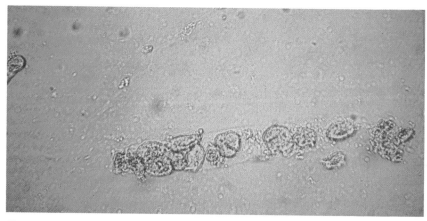

Figure 29

Hyaline casts are pale, colorless, occasionally refractile "cylinders". They are best seen when the intensity of the light is sharply reduced. These casts are formed of the gel of proteins which have presumably traversed the glomerular capillary membrane. (Figure 30)

HYALINE CAST, High power

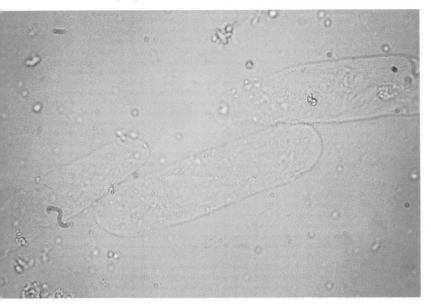

Figure 30

CRYSTALS

A variety of crystals may appear in the urine. These can be identified by their specific appearances and solubility characteristics, (Table 6).

The crystals normally found in acid urine are the yellow-red granular urates, octahedral or envelope-shaped calcium oxalate and the yellow or red-brown irregularly-shaped, rhomboidal wedge, prism, or rossette-shaped uric acid crystals. Dumbbell-shaped calcium carbonate and large, colorless, prism-shaped triple phosphate crystals occur in alkaline urine.

Most crystal are nonpathological. Some, however, indicate pathology. Cystine crystals (Figure 31) are indicative of cystinuria, a condition in which cystine stones form in the kidney, and cystinosis, an inborn error of metabolism in which cystine crystals are found in the urine, reticuloendothelial system, spleen and eyes.

85

HEXAGONAL CYSTINE CRYSTALS, High power

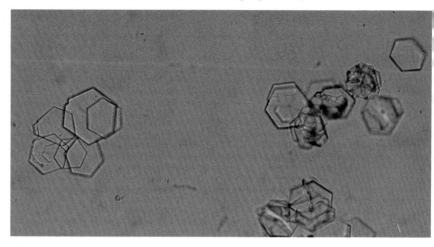

Figure 31

Uric acid crystals may appear in the urine, in a variety of shapes and color. They may appear as a result of pathology or as a result of normal metabolism. Uric acid may appear as needles, hexagonal shape, rosette shape, "whetstone form", or as rhombic plates. Crystals may appear colorless, yellow or brown. Increased uric acid denotes increased purine metabolism and uric acid crystals may be found in cases of fever, leukemia, some renal tubular diseases, and gout. Figure 32 shows uric acid crystals.

URIC ACID, High power

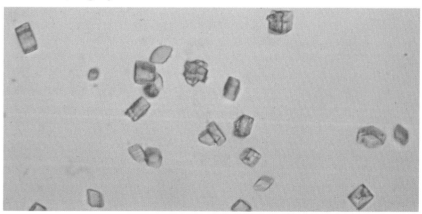

Figure 32

86

Leucine and tyrosine are abnormal crystal occasionally seen in urine of patients with liver problems. When there are severe liver problems, these aminoacids are not metabolized. Tyrosine crystals appear as colorless fine needles and are usually grouped in clusters. (Figure 33)

TYROSINE, High power

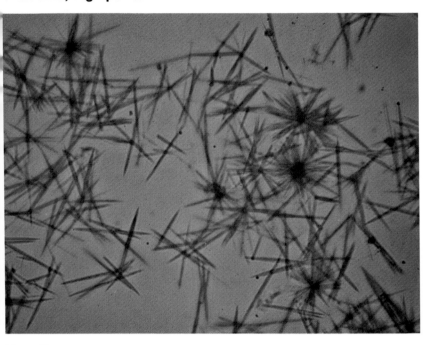

Figure 33

Drug crystals are not normally found in random urine. Occasionally "sulfa" crystals may be seen in acid urine of patients who do not hydrate correctly by drinking enough water. The sulfa drugs produced recently are very soluble compounds and sulfa crystals are not frequently found in urine.

BACTERIA

Bacteria may be seen in the sediment as a result of either urinary tract infection or contamination of the specimen. The two causes cannot usually be distinguished by examination of the sediment, although the presence of large numbers of leucocytes with a positive nitrite, is suggestive of urinary tract infection. Bacilli are more easily recognized than cocci, which may be mistaken for amorphous crystals. A culture should be performed when in doubt. (Figure 34)

BACTERIA, High power

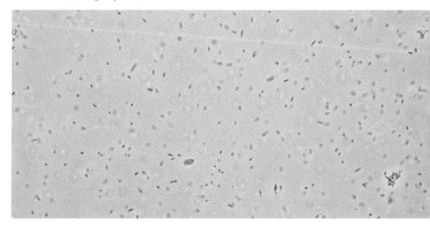

Figure 34

YEAST

Yeast cells may be seen in the urinary sediment. They are sometimes confused with red blood cells. They differ by being ovoid rather than round, colorless, variable in size and frequently may show budding. If in doubt, the addition of acetic acid will lyse red blood cells but leave yeast cells intact. Large amounts of yeast with hyphae are suggestive of vaginitis. (Figure 35)

YEAST, High power

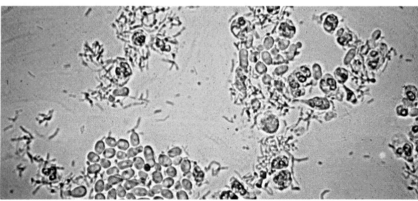

Figure 35

PARASITES

Trichomonas vaginalis is the most frequently seen parasite in urine. It is a unicellular organism with anterior flagellae and undulating membrane. In appearance, the parasite may resemble flattened, ovoid epithelial cells but are usually recognized by their swimming motions through the sediment and the movements of its flagellates and the characteristic undulating membrane. (Figure 36)

TRICHOMONAS VAGINALIS, High power

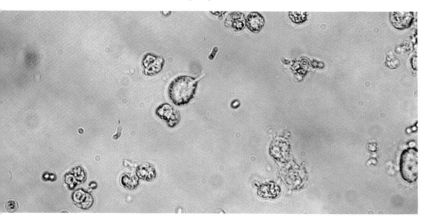

Figure 36

SPERMATOZOA

Spermatozoa have oval bodies long delicate tails. They may be motile or stationary. (Figure 37)

SPERMATOZOA, High power

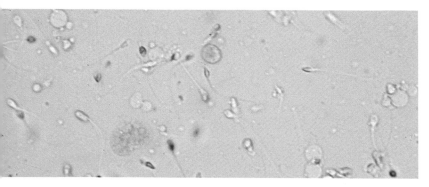

Figure 37.

CONTAMINANTS AND ARTIFACTS

Cotton threads, hair, starch granules, wood and wool fibers, and other contaminants must be recognized adequately enough to ascertain that these substances do not represent any significant finding in the urinary sediment. An example of cotton fibers and starch granules are shown below.

COTTON FIBERS, Low power

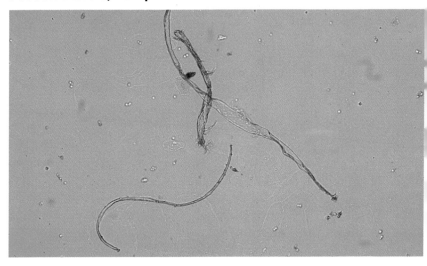

Figure 38.

STARCH GRANULES, High power

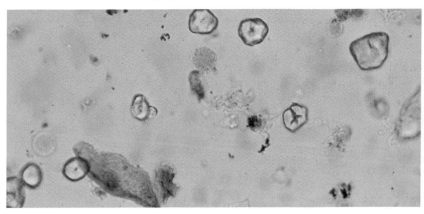

Figure 39.

90

QUANTITATIVE EVALUATION OF THE URINE SEDIMENT—THE ADDIS COUNT

The Addis count is a quantitative measurement of the excretion of red blood cells, leucocytes, and casts in the urine during a 12 hour period. Protein excretion during the same time period and the specific gravity of the sample can also be determined.

Reference Values

Normal values for all of these parameters have been established. Red blood cell excretion normally does not exceed 500,000 per 12 hours, leucocyte excretion is no greater than 1,000,000 per 12 hours, and the excretion of hyaline casts is equal to or less than 5,000 per 12 hours. Normal protein excretion should not exceed 0.150 gm. per 24 hours, and normal specific gravity, indicative of adequate concentrating ability, is 1.025 or higher.

Values in Disease States

Increased excretion of red blood cells, leucocytes, and casts usually occurs in the urine of patients with glomerulonephritis. The rates of excretion of these elements reflect the degree of activity of the disease and thus indicate the severity of the renal disorder. Since the numbers of red blood cells, leucocytes, and casts are measured for a specific period of time, comparisons can be made of the rates of excretion of these elements during the course of a specific disease and in relation to established norms of excretion of these elements for the same disease.

Procedure

A timed overnight urine specimen is obtained in the following manner: the patient is not permitted to ingest fluids after lunch on the day before the test. The patient voids prior to bedtime, notes the exact time of voiding, and discards the urine. Upon arising, the patient voids all urine into a collection bottle that contains formalin preservative, and notes the exact time of voiding.

In the laboratory this timed specimen is mixed thoroughly and then measured accurately in a graduated cylinder. A drop of caprylic alcohol is added to the cylinder to prevent foaming. A volume of urine equal to the amount excreted in 12 minutes (1/5 hour) is determined by calculation based on knowledge of total volume and total time of collection or through the use of a nomogram specific for this determination. This amount, if it equals 15 ml or less, is centrifuged for 5 minutes at 1750 to 2000 rpm. If the 12 minute volume is greater than 15 ml, half the amount (a 6-minute volume) is taken and a correction factor is used later in the calculations. After centrifugation, the supernatant fluid is withdrawn until exactly 0.5 ml remains. The supernatant fluid may be used for quantitative protein determination. The sediment in the centrifuge tube is completely resuspended in the remaining 0.5 ml left in the tube and a sufficient number of drops of this suspension are used to fill a standard hemocytometer counting chamber.

Casts are counted under low power magnification as the number of casts in six adjacent large squares (1 × 1 mm each). Red blood cells are counted under high power (dry) magnification as the number of cells in 13 adjacent medium-sized squares. The combined leucocytes and epithelial cells are counted in the same way. The counting procedure should be repeated up to 10 times, using the average number of cells and casts per count for the remaining calculations.

The average number of casts per six squares is multiplied by 100,000 to equal the number of casts excreted in 24 hours or by 50,000 to equal the number excreted in 12 hours. The average number of red cells, and the average number of leucocytes and epithelial cells per 13 squares is multiplied by 100,000 to determine the number of cells excreted in 24 hours, or by 500,000 for the number excreted in 12 hours. When the original volume centrifuged is equal to six minutes (1/10 hour) of urine formation, each of the results as calculated above must be doubled.

QUALITATIVE DESCRIPTION OF URINARY SEDIMENT VERSUS THE ADDIS COUNT

A qualitative description of the urinary sediment, although subject to the errors of a variable concentration of urine, is most useful for the general diagnosis of renal disease. The Addis count, or specific quantitation of excreted red blood cells, leucocytes, epithelial cells, and casts in the urine, is most useful in evaluating the course of a given disease. The Addis count cannot replace the qualitative examination of the urinary sediment as it serves an entirely different function. Moreover, it is a time-consuming technique, both in collection of the specimen and in the determination performed in the laboratory. The possibility of errors in calculation are great as the multiplication factors are very large and a slight error in the number of cells or casts counted can make a difference of several million cells or casts in the estimated excretion rate. Table 8 shows a comparison of the Addis count and routine urine sediment examination.

Table 8

A COMPARISON OF ADDIS COUNTS AND ROUTINE EXAMINATION OF THE SEDIMENT

FORMED ELEMENT	SEMI-QUANTITATIVE (ADDIS COUNT TOTAL EXCRETION PER 12 HOURS)	ROUTINE SCREENING EXAMINATION (PER HIGH-POWER-FIELD)
	6,700 to 79,000	0 or 1—2
Casts	122,000 to 1,000,000	1—2
	6,000,000 to 15,000,000	10—20
	220,000 to 2,400,000	0—10
Red Cells	2,500,000 to 8,200,000	1—20
	190,000,000 to 570,000,000	5—60
	Less than 1,000,000	0 (occasionally) 3—5 (usually) 10—20 (rare)
Leukocytes and Epithelial cells	1,000,000 to 10,000,000	5—10
	10,000,000 to 75,000,000	10—20 (clumped)

CONTROLS

19.

The use of controls in the clinical laboratory has been in wide practice for many years. Controls provide the laboratory professional with the capability to evaluate the changes and/or errors that are commonly associated with routine clinical chemistry. The controls should be used to establish confidence that the variables which cause errors are in check or within a range of acceptability as established by the laboratory. Guidelines have been established to aid the laboratory to initiate a quality control program using solutions of known values. By understanding the trends established by responsible interpretation of control values, better results are obtained with clinical procedures.

Controls are tested often, usually in duplicate, in routine chemical assays of serum simply to control laboratory error.

Urinalysis is not so fortunate, even though there are more errors which may cause unreliable results. Relatively few laboratories use controls in urine chemistry because of lack of apparent need. Some reasons given for not using controls are:

1. Strips are "read" visually.
2. Results are subjective.
3. Urinalysis results are not important.
4. Strips are simple.
5. No standard used, so no need for control.

Of course, all of the above statements indicate need for control in urinalysis because more variables exist. Examine each parameter.

1. Strips may be read or interpreted visually by judging the difference in color change as referenced against a negative color block. Color interpretation with urine chemistry reagent strips is perhaps the most subjective determination in the clinical laboratory. Everyone "reads" color differently. There is considerable variation from person to person and laboratory to laboratory. This is an excellent reason, if not the single most important reason, to have and use controls in urinalysis.

2. The colors the eyes "see" need to be controlled and uniform so interpretation can be made without large numbers of additional variables. New instrumentation such as the CLINI-TEK® and CLINILAB® were designed specifically to correct the problems listed above.

3. Urinalysis results are not important. This is not true, of course, and routine urinalysis is done virtually everywhere. More clinical data is obtained with urine than all other body fluids combined. The variability of results reported can be "controlled", thus making clinical results more meaningful.
4. Strips are simple. To use, they are, but in chemical principle they are not. The chemical interaction is as complicated, if not more so, than the wet chemical test to which they are referenced.
5. No "standard" is used, so no need for controls. The standard in reagent strip urinalysis is the color chart. By comparing the degree of positiveness to a "standard" color, interpretation can be made. Color cannot be memorized, so comparisons using proper timing, in good lighting, must be made. More variables are eliminated , thus, better results are obtained.

Quality control brings into check variables that occur in any procedure. The degree of control is usually established by the laboratory. Outside agencies and professional organizations have also suggested that controls be used in urinalysis.

Controls should be tested at least once per day, when new reagents are used, or when clinical results are in question. By using a negative and composite positive (CHEK-STIX®) as knowns, confidence that no "false positives" are obtained increases. The positive control gives confidence that Ames urinalysis reagents are reacting properly with positive specimens. A hidden control also provides evidence that proper handling and testing procedures are being followed. All results should be recorded on a quality control chart. Urinalysis is slipping out of control if a negative urine is called a positive more than 5% of the time for any individual reagent area and/or a positive reaction is called a negative more than 5% of the time on any of the areas of Ames reagent strips.

CONCLUSION

The performance of controls in urinalysis is an important part of the total urinalysis and clinical chemistry picture. Interpretation of control results is essential, even though routine. The greatest single problem in an effective program is that technicians learn to ignore control charts even though they are actually keeping them up to date. When the quality control program has been established, its value will be lost completely if the need for action indicated by its results is ignored.

By realizing that quality control assesses the sources of variables, from specimen transporting to recording of results, better values are obtained—not necessarily the perfect value, but a result obtained with a high degree of confidence in procedures used.

APPENDIX I

TABLE OF AVERAGE NORMAL VALUES FOR URINE DETERMINATIONS*

TEST	AVERAGE NORMAL VALUE	TYPE OF SPECIMEN
Addis Count	wbc 1,800,000 rbc 500,000 casts 0-5,000	12 hour

Albumin
  qualitative
  quantitative
Aldosterone
	
	negative
	10-100 mg/24 hr
	2-23 μg/24 hour
		
		random
		24 hour
		24 hour, refrigerated

Amino acid nitrogen	100-290 mg/24 hour	24 hour, refrigerated collected in thymol
Ammonia	20-70 mEq/24 hr	24 hour
Ammonia nitrogen	0.14-1.47 gm/24 hr	24 hour
Bence Jones Protein	negative	first morning specimen
Bilirubin	negative	random
Blood, occult	negative	random

Calcium
  Sulkowitch
  quantitative
	
	positive 1+
	100-250 mg/24 hr
	on an average diet
		
		random
		24 hour

Catecholamines	100-230 μg/24 hr	24 hour, preserve with 1 ml. concentrated H_2SO_4
Chloride	110-250 mEq/24 hr	24 hour
Concentration test	Specific gravity of 1.025 or higher	Withholding fluids for the day prior to the test

Coproporphyrin
  random
  24 hour
	20 μg/100 ml
	adults
	  50-200 μg/24 hr
	children:
	  0-80 μg/24 hr
		random
		24 hour, preserve with 5 gm. Na_2CO_3

Creatine	male:
	  0-40 mg/24 hr
	female:
	  0-100 mg/24 hr
	higher in children
		24 hour

TEST	AVERAGE NORMAL VALUE	TYPE OF SPECIMEN

Creatinine	male:
	  1.0-1.9 gm/24 hr
	female:
	  0.8-1.7 gm/24 hr
		24 hour

Dilution test	Specific gravity of 1.001 to 1.003	After 1200 ml water load

Estrogens	male:
	  4-25 μg/24 hr
	female:
	  4-60 μg/24 hr
		24 hour, refrigerate

Glucose
  qualitative
  quantitative
	
	negative
	130 mg/24 hr
		
		random
		24 hour

Hemoglobin	negative	random

17-hydroxycortico-
  steroids
	
	males:
	  5.5-14.5 mg/24 hr
	females:
	  5-13 mg/24 hr
		
		24 hour, tranquilizers
		interfere

17-ketosteroids	males:
	  8-15 mg/24 hr
	females:
	  6-11.5 mg/24 hr
	children:
	  5 mg/24 hr
		24 hour, tranquilizers
		interfere

Ketones	negative	random
Lead	100 μg/24 hr	24 hour, collect in lead-free bottle

Osmolality
  Normal fluid intake
  full range
	
	500-800 mOsm/kg water
	38-1400 mOsm/kg water
		
		random
		random

pH	4.6-8.0	random
Phenylpyruvic acid	negative	random
Phosphorus	0.9-1.3 gm/24 hr	24 hour
Porphobilinogen	negative	random
Potassium	25-100 mEq/24 hr	24 hour

Pregnanediol	male:
	  0-1 mg/24 hr
	female:
	  1-8 mg/24 hr
	children:
	  negative
		24 hour, refrigerate

TEST	AVERAGE NORMAL VALUE	TYPE OF SPECIMEN
Pregnanetriol	male: 1.0-2.0 mg/24 hr female: 0.5-2.0 mg/24 hr children: <0.5 mg/24 hr.	24 hour, refrigerate
Protein qualitative quantitative Bence Jones	negative 10-150 mg/24 hr negative	random 24 hour first morning specimen
Sodium	110-260 mEq/24 hr	24 hour
Specific gravity random 24-hour	1.002-1.030 1.015-1.025	random 24 hour
Sugars	negative	random
Titratable acidity	200-500 ml of 0.1 N NaOH/24 hr	24 hour, preserve with toluene
Urea nitrogen	6-17 gm/24 hr	24 hour
Uric acid	250-750 mg/24 hr	24 hour
Urobilinogen semiquantitative quantitative	0.3-1.0 Ehrlich units/2 hr 1.0-4.0 mg/24 hr	2 hour afternoon specimen 24 hour, collect in dark bottle with 5 gm Na_2CO_3, refrigerate
Uroporphyrin	10-30 μg/24 hr	24 hour, collect in dark bottle with 5 gm Na_2CO_3
VMA (Vanilmandelic acid)	1-8 mg/24 hr	24 hour, preserve in 3 ml. 25% H_2SO_4. No coffee or fruit for 2 days prior to test.
Volume adults	600-1500 ml/24 hr	24 hour

*After Davidsohn, I. and Henry, J. B., *Todd-Sanford Clinical Diagnosis by Laboratory Methods*, W. B. Saunders Company, Philadelphia, 1969, and Goodale, R. H. and Widmann, F. K., *Clinical Interpretation of Laboratory Tests*, F. A. Davis Company, Philadelphia, 1969.

APPENDIX II

TABLE OF RAPID REAGENT TESTS FOR ROUTINE AND SPECIAL URINALYSIS

Findings obtained by urinalysis provide the physician with an extensive amount of important information regarding the status of the individual patient's health. Much of this information is obtained quickly, conveniently, and reliably by using modern reagent strips and tablets without need for specialized equipment and complex procedures. The following table shows the wide range of Ames reagent strips and tablets that are readily available for use.

Of these, N-MULTISTIX®-SG, which provides nine clinically significant findings from a urine specimen, is undoubtedly the most useful method for routine urinalysis. Other reagent strips and tests are frequently useful when special tests are requested.

MICROSTIX®-3, the 3-way bacterial test, can expand the services of a urinalysis laboratory by providing information useful to the physician for confirming a clinical diagnosis of urinary tract infection, for follow-up testing 48 hours or more after cessation of therapy, and for early detection of significant asymptomatic bacteriuria in high-risk patients.

REAGENT TEST	SUBSTANCES DETERMINED	VISUAL TECHNIQUE*
N-MULTISTIX®	pH, protein, glucose, acetoacetic acid, bilirubin, blood, nitrite and urobilinogen	Use fresh, uncentrifuged urine. Certain preservatives may be added. Dip reagent strip in specimen, remove, and compare each reagent area with corresponding color chart on bottle label at the number of seconds specified.
N-MULTISTIX-C®	pH, protein, glucose, acetoacetic acid, bilirubin, blood, nitrite, urobilinogen and ascorbic acid	as above
N-MULTISTIX®-SG	pH, protein, glucose, acetoacetic acid, bilirubin, blood, nitrite, urobilinogen and specific gravity	as above

REAGENT TEST	SUBSTANCES DETERMINED	VISUAL TECHNIQUE*
MULTISTIX®	pH, protein, glucose, acetoacetic acid, bilirubin, blood, and urobilinogen	as above
BILI-LABSTIX®	pH, protein, glucose, acetoacetic acid, bilirubin, and blood	as above
LABSTIX®	pH, protein, glucose, acetoacetic acid, and blood	as above
HEMA-COMBISTIX®	pH, protein, glucose, and blood	as above
COMBISTIX®	pH, protein and glucose	as above
N-URISTIX®	protein, glucose and nitrite	as above
URISTIX®	protein and glucose	as above
CLINISTIX®	glucose	as above
ALBUSTIX®	protein	as above
HEMASTIX®	blood	as above
MICROSTIX® NITRITE	nitrite	as above
UROBILISTIX®	urobilinogen	as above, but preferably using a 2 hour urine specimen collected in early afternoon (between 2 and 4 P.M.)
MICROSTIX®-3	bacteriuria	Dip culture-reagent strip in specimen for 5 seconds, remove, read nitrite test area after 30 seconds. Insert and seal strip in sterilized plastic pouch provided, incubate for 18 to 24 hours. Compare color densities on total and Gram-negative culture pads with chart provided, without removing strip from pouch. Incinerate pouch with strip still sealed inside.
ICTOTEST®	bilirubin	Place 5 drops of urine on the special mat. Cover with the reagent tablet. Flow 2 drops of water onto the tablet. Compare the color reaction with the color chart.

REAGENT TEST	SUBSTANCES DETERMINED	VISUAL TECHNIQUE*
DIASTIX®	glucose	Use fresh, uncentrifuged urine. Do not use preservative containing formaldehyde. Dip reagent strip in specimen, remove, and compare with color chart on bottle label.
KETOSTIX®	acetoacetic acid	As above, but urine must be at least at room temperature at the time of testing.
KETO-DIASTIX®	glucose and aceto-acetic acid	as above for DIASTIX and KETOSTIX.
CLINITEST®	reducing substances, including sugars	Add CLINITEST tablet to test tube containing mixture of 5 drops of urine and 10 drops of water. Spontaneous boiling occurs; after it stops, compare color in tube with color chart. Alternate method uses 2 drops of urine and 2 drop color chart.
PHENISTIX®	phenylpyruvic acid (phenylketonuria, or PKU)	Use fresh, uncentrifuged urine. Dip reagent strip in specimen, remove, and compare with color chart on bottle label.

*See package inserts for proper procedures. CLINI-TEK® Reagents are chemically the same as the visual strips. The CLINI-TEK® strips have a special reflectance chip which allow them to be read by the CLINI-TEK®.

SELECTED REFERENCES

1. Addis, T. *Glomerular Nephritis: Diagnosis and Treatment,* The Macmillan Company, 1949.
2. Allen A. C. *The Kidney: Medical and Surgical Diseases,* 2nd edition, Grune and Stratton, 1962.
3. Brody, L. H., Salladay, J. R., and Armbruster, K. Urinalysis and the Urinary Sediment, *Medical Clinics of North America, 55:*243, 1971.
4. Brunnell, P. A., ed. Symposium on Laboratory Diagnosis, *Pediatric Clinics of North America 18:* No. 1, February 1971.
5. Davidsohn, I. and Henry J. B. *Todd-Sanford Clinical Diagnosis by Labratory Methods,* 14th edition, W. B. Saunders Company, 1969.
6. Frankel, S., Reitman, S. and Sonnenworth, A. C. *Gradwohl's Clinical Laboratory Methods and Diagnosis,* Vol. 2, 6th edition, The C. V. Mosby Company, 1963.
7. Freake, R. and Nayman, J. *Atlas of Urinary Deposits,* Melbourne University Press, 1969.
8. Goodale, R. H. and Widmann, F. K. *Clinical Interpretation of Laboratory Tests,* 6th edition, F. A. Davis Company, 1969.
9. Ham T. H. *A Syllabus of Laboratory Examinations in Clinical Diagnosis,* Harvard University Press, 1956.
10. Harrison, T. R., Adams, R. D., Bennett, I. L., Resnik, W. H. Thorn, G. W., and Wintrabe, M. N. *Principles of Internal Medicine,* 4th edition, McGraw-Hill Book Company, Inc., 1962.
11. Hsia, D. Y-Y. *Inborn Errors of Metabolism, Part I. Clinical Aspects.* 2nd edition, Year Book Medical Publishers, Inc., 1966.
12. Hsia, D. Y-Y. and Inouya, T. *Inborn Errors of Metabolism, Part 2. Laboratory Methods,* Year Book Medical Publishers, Inc., 1966.
13. James, J. A. *Renal Disease in Childhood,* The C. V. Mosby Company, 1968.
14. Jawetz, E., Melnick, J. L. and Adelberg, E. A. *Review of Medical Microbiology,* 2nd edition, Lange Medical Publications, 1956.
15. Kark, R. M., Lawrence, J. R. Pollak, V. E., Pirani, C. L., Muehrcke, R. C., and Silva, H. *A Primer of Urinalysis,* 2nd edition, Hoeber Medical Division, 1963.
16. Kark, R. M., ed. Symposium on Diseases of the Kidney, *Medical Clinics of North America* Vol. 55, No. 1, January 1971.
17. Kolmer, J. A. *Clinical Diagnosis by Laboratory Examinations,* 3rd edition, Appelton-Century-Crofts, Inc., 1961.
18. Levinson, S. A. and MacFate, R. P. *Clinical Laboratory Diagnosis,* 7th edition, Lea and Febiger, 1969.
19. Lippman, R. W. *Urine and the Urinary Sediment. A Practical Manual and Atlas,* 2nd edition, Charles C. Thomas, 1957.
20. Merrill, J. P. *The Treatment of Renal Failure,* Grune and Stratton, 1955.
21. Page, L. B. and Culver P. J. *A Syllabus of Laboratory Examinations in Clinical Diagnosis,* Harvard University Press, 1961.
22. Pitts, R. F. *Physiology of the Kidney and Body Fluids,* Year Book Medical Publishers, Inc., 1963.
23. Reubi, F. C. *Clearance Tests in Clinical Medicine,* Charles C. Thomas, 1963.
24. Smith H. W. *Principles of Renal Physiology,* Oxford University Press, 1956.
25. Smith, H. W. *The Kidney, Structure and Function in Health and Disease,* Oxford University Press, 1951.
26. Strauss, M. B. and Welt, L. G. *Diseases of the Kidney,* Little, Brown and Co. 1963.
27. Sunderman, F. W. and Sunderman, F. W. Jr. *Laboratory Diagnosis of Kidney Disease,* Warren H. Green, Inc., 1970.
28. Wilson, G. S. and Miles, A. A. *Topley and Wilson's Principles of Bacteriology and Immunology,* 4th edition, The Williams and Wilkins Co., 1955.
29. Wolman, J. J. *Laboratory Applications in Clinical Pediatrics,* The Blakiston Division, 1957.